LOOKING BACK TO NOW:
A MEMOIR

MEARA NIGRO

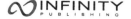

ISBN: 978-1-4958-2065-6 Paperback
ISBN: 978-1-4958-2066-3 Hardcover
ISBN: 978-1-4958-2067-0 eBook
Library of Congress Control Number: 2017-913822

Looking Back to Now is a memoir.

Published October 2017

INFINITY PUBLISHING
1094 New DeHaven Street, Suite 100
West Conshohocken, PA 19428-2713
Toll-free (877) BUY BOOK
Local Phone (610) 941-9999
Fax (610) 941-9959
Info@buybooksontheweb.com
www.buybooksontheweb.com

DEDICATION PAGE:

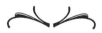

To my husband Bruce whose devotion took us to Ireland, Croatia, Montenegro, Denmark, Norway, Montana, Nevada and parts of the Oregon-California Trail so that I could write this book.

1

Sam died the other day. At first, I didn't even notice he wasn't sitting in his usual spot – the flowered sofa by the window. I only discovered he had died because my eyes were drawn to a photo of a bride and groom on a table by the fireplace so I took a closer look to see if the bride was someone on the staff. That's when I noticed the picture of Sam next to the wedding photo with the handwritten message, "Our friend Sam passed on. He will be missed by staff and residents alike."

I hadn't even known his name was Sam. I just knew him as the other half of "the Couple." Sam and his lady friend Aggie met at Rose Hall Assisted Living. She was 100 and he was 95. They always sat on the flowered sofa together, holding hands and alternately taking naps. Usually, it was Aggie who was asleep. Sometimes, as I walked by on my way to my mother's apartment, they would both be awake at the same time, but I never caught them both asleep.

Sam was the more outgoing of the two. He began to recognize me as a regular, his face brightening into a broad smile and he'd give me a jaunty wave as I passed by the sofa. I'd call out, "Good morning!" and wave back.

One day, as I passed by and Aggie was napping by his side, Sam blew a string of kisses ending with a rakish grin. I felt oddly pleased, realizing that to Sam's 95-year-old eyes, I was a hot young babe even though I'd been a member of AARP for many years.

Ivy, the live-in aide I recently hired, answered the door. My mother was dressed in her new pants suit that I had managed to sneak into her wardrobe now that she no longer remembered she abhorred slacks on women. Slacks are warmer and the kind of dresses that she has preferred all these years no longer seem to be available anywhere. So with her mind almost a clean slate, except for everything that happened before 1937, I was able to convince her she'd be right in style and much more comfortable in the winter.

She hadn't heard my knock on the door. Her head was slumped over and little noises, half-way between a cat's purr and the wind whistling down the chimney, came from her throat. It used to scare me when I saw her like this, but now I knew her body just shut down at intervals throughout the day to conserve her energy. I touched her shoulder gently and crooned, "Hellooo, it's me. I'm here to take you out."

Her eyes opened and instantly her face was transformed by a radiant grin. "Oh, you're here. I was hoping you'd come."

I had called not a half-hour before to tell her I was on my way, and still my visit was a complete surprise.

Other times, when I gently shook her awake from her nap, she'd look at me with eyes wide and exclaim, "Good heavens! I haven't seen you in years." On those occasions, I knew she thought I was her dear friend Katherine from Butte, Montana. Ten minutes later, she would call me by my name and introduce me to other residents as her daughter and by the end of our visit, she'd be reminiscing about our childhood together in Butte. It was easiest on both of us if I just entered her reality and went along for the ride. Correcting her was pointless and only added to her feelings of inadequacy and depression.

The first time this happened, she was 88 and still living on her own in the house in Metuchen where I grew up. She seemed to be doing very well and it wasn't that long ago that I had been bragging to people that my 84-year-old mother was still working full-time because she couldn't stand the thought of having nothing to do.

Retirement couldn't be avoided forever, though. The doctor she had worked for since he opened his Ob/Gyn practice in 1952 was loyal and patient. But when he retired, the younger doctors who took over the practice eased her out.

It was Thanksgiving and my son Jay was going to swing by her house and pick her up. Then she called in tears because she couldn't find her keys so she wouldn't be able to leave her house, literally, because all her doors had deadbolts that were locked from the inside. She wouldn't have been able to open the doors to leave even if her life depended on it.

Years ago, fortunately, my mother had given me a set of keys to her house so the day was saved and we were able to bring her over to my house for the holiday. After dinner, Mom and my daughter Dana and I sat in the living room while my husband Bruce and Jay caught up on football scores. Mom turned to me and asked, "Were you here during the Depression or were you still living in Europe at the time?"

The question, coming out of nowhere like that, struck me as funny and I laughed. "I wasn't even born yet. I was born in 1946," I answered.

Startled, she looked as though she wanted to disown the words out of her own mouth. She clamped her lips shut and looked around, apparently grateful there had been only two witnesses to her gaffe. When I looked at Dana, there were tears in her eyes. Seeing this sudden change in her grandmother was very upsetting, while I, for some perverse reason, found it amusing. This was just the beginning of that long passage between generations that many families go through if the elderly parents only live long enough. My own grandparents had died long before I was born and my husband's parents had died in their fifties so we were novices in the skill that's required in learning how to parent one's own parent, especially one as strong-willed and independent as my mother.

She could be a formidable woman. At least that's how I had always felt about her until I was well into my fifties and finally had enough gumption to stand up to her. Gumption was something she approved of and when I displayed it in any situation other than in defying her, she was proud. She often said I was the only one in our family who *had* gumption, but we locked horns when I could no longer avoid dealing with her increasing frailty and mental confusion.

My brother Mark and I developed a plan to keep her in her own house as long as possible. He would spend two nights a week there, arriving around midnight after his shift at *The Record* was over. They'd have breakfast together and he'd take her grocery shopping or help her run any other errands she needed done in an effort to cut down on the number of times she ventured out alone in her car. Bruce and I would take her out for Sunday breakfast, her favorite meal of the day, make a stop at the ATM, a magical machine to my mother, and then maybe go to the park for a little walk. Back at her house, one of us would keep her busy in the kitchen while the other one went through her desk to see if important mail was piling up and bills weren't being paid. Eventually, it became necessary to create a living trust to pay all her bills because paranoia was making her suspicious of us.

During Mark's visits, he'd cook a few meals and put them in the refrigerator so she could just reheat them in the evening. I would call her every day from work to chat and make sure she was all right. She was delighted to hear from me and would sometimes exclaim, to my dismay, "You're the only person I've spoken to all day!" She would often sound out of breath and say she had been doing laundry in the basement or was cleaning the kitchen. I would sometimes ask what she'd had for dinner and she'd assure me she'd eaten a delicious piece of chicken, a baked potato and some vegetables. But then when we'd show up on Sunday, she'd often be wearing the same soiled dress she had on the last time I saw her and the meals that Mark had carefully prepared for her earlier in the week were still in the refrigerator. Increasingly, it became apparent that chicken or a pork chop did not appeal to her as much as Hägen Dazs ice cream or candy.

At this point, she still had her car and would drive to the A&P a few times a week. We hated to deprive her of this little bit of freedom because it was the last vestige of independence and contact with the outside world on her terms, and to be honest, we didn't have courage enough yet to face her wrath if we took her car away. The highlight of her day would be encountering someone she knew as she pushed her grocery cart up and down each aisle. We were thankful she knew her reflexes were not adequate to deal with busy traffic patterns or pedestrians suddenly charging out into the street so she went out only at mid-day when children were in school and she avoided roads that required left-hand turns without a traffic light.

But then, one day as she slowly pulled into the A&P parking lot, a man waved her over and told her there was something wrong with one of her tires. He offered to take a look at it, and because my mother had never encountered anyone before who would do her harm, she was grateful for his gentlemanly offer of help. He tinkered with the wheel for a few minutes and then told her he could fix it with a simple part that would cost about $40. My mother checked her wallet and found she had only $30 in it, but she assured the man that she had more money at home. He offered to follow her home and she could pay him there. The story could have had a tragic ending, but thankfully the man only wanted quick cash. As she reached into the desk drawer where she kept extra money, he pushed her aside, took the handful of twenties from her most recent visit to the ATM and ran out of the house. My mother was shaken and distraught, but she didn't call the police *or* me. Somehow, in her growing mental confusion, I had become someone who couldn't be trusted, perhaps because I had suggested that moving to an assisted living facility or hiring a live-in aide would be a good idea. She did confide in Mark who she regarded as her ally.

She also confided to him that I had stolen her emerald engagement ring and the family silver. I was devastated that she really seemed to believe I had stolen the ring she had given to me when arthritis made it impossible to fit it over her swollen fingers. And she had given her parents' silver flatware and serving pieces to me when she could no longer host the holidays and my home became the center of family gatherings.

Her doctor ordered some tests and prescribed a new drug that was supposed to help slow the progression of dementia. At times she understood that her memory loss had probably been caused by a series of little strokes - in other words, an illness that wasn't her fault. But more often, she just felt stupid and couldn't understand why recalling things that had once been easy for her now verged on the impossible. "Sometimes," she confided to me one day, "I feel like a character in a book I haven't read yet."

But she had never been a dependent woman so accepting these new and painful limitations caused her to alternately lash out at us or to retreat into depression. She refused to move from her home to an assisted living facility or to allow a person she didn't know move in with her. She wouldn't even allow me to hire a cleaning woman once a week to help her even though her three-story house with five bedrooms was too much for an 89-year-old woman to maintain, and her bathroom was on the second floor, necessitating far too many perilous trips up and down the stairs.

As a compromise, she bought one of those gadgets she could wear around her neck so she could press a button to alert the local authorities if she needed help. I was very pleased until I discovered she wasn't wearing the gadget because she didn't want strangers bashing her door in. "But what if you're lying at the foot of the stairs with a broken hip? You'll be in agony and won't be able to reach the phone to call for help," I protested. I implored her to have a second bathroom installed downstairs so she could sleep in the dining room if the day ever came when stairs were too much for her. "I hope I'm dead by then," was her usual response and that was the end of the discussion.

She had planned very well for her old age, investing her salary as an office manager/bookkeeper in a variety of stocks and bonds that had grown steadily over the years, and because she had continued working long past the age when most people retire, she could save her bigger-than-average Social Security checks. When long-term care insurance became available, she was one of the first to buy it. She had visited her lawyer regularly to keep her will up to date and drafted a living will to make sure everyone understood she wanted no heroic measures taken to keep her alive at the end. She took the initiative in arranging for me to have Power of Attorney and made me come to her bank once a year to introduce me to everyone, as an extra precaution. She wrote down all her instructions and made us sit through periodic reviews of them so we would know what to do when she died, including having me go to the funeral home with her to discuss her pre-paid arrangements so the funeral director would know that *I* knew she didn't want me being shamed into paying for a more extravagant funeral than what she planned. My mother had a no-nonsense practicality about death and her primary fear was slipping into a long, slow decline in a nursing home, wasting all her hard-earned money.

In her early 80's, back before dementia started taking its toll, my mother tried to make me promise I would kill her if she ever got to the point where she couldn't take care of herself. "I can't do that," I protested. "I don't even like to kill bugs. I catch mice in a HavaHart® trap and let them go outside. I can't kill my own mother!"

"What good are you?" she said with obvious disgust. Trying to reason with her, I said I'd end up spending the rest of my life in prison, thinking she wouldn't want that to be my fate, or short of that, she wouldn't want the public scandal.

"That won't happen, if you do it right," was her tart reply.

I've lost count of how many times over the next few years that we had this discussion. Finally, by the time she was 89, my brother and I couldn't avoid the truth. Allowing her to continue living alone with her stairs, deadbolts, electrical cords stretching across rooms, stove knobs that turned the gas on as she brushed by them and a childlike willingness to admit to telemarketers on the phone that she lived all alone would be like allowing a three-year-old to live without any adult supervision.

Bruce and I told her as gently as we could that it was necessary to move to Rose Hall, a lovely assisted living facility near us that would, in many respects, seem like being on vacation. It looked very much like a gracious country inn with good food, entertainment, interesting activities, a hair salon, and she could have her own furniture in her apartment. We had visited the place and were very impressed.

She looked around the living room of the house she had lived in for 54 years, the home where she had raised her children and where a lifetime of memories were housed and began to cry. Then I began to cry. Perhaps sensing a weakening in my resolve, she begged me to kill her rather than force her to move to a strange place.

Watching this drama unfold, Bruce stepped in and said, "But she won't go to heaven if she kills you." My mother stopped crying and looked first at him, then at me. I never knew this intensely practical woman who hadn't been to church in several decades even believed in heaven, but the idea that her daughter would be forever locked out of paradise, and might actually be doomed to spending eternity in hell, settled the issue.

At least it settled that I was not willing to kill her, but she still vacillated dramatically on the issue of moving to assisted living. She surprised us one day by agreeing quite cheerfully to visit the facility with Bruce and me and seemed impressed with all the amenities designed to make life more comfortable. She especially liked the receptionist's cute little dog and the walk-in bathtub that struck her as a marvelously ingenious invention so she sat down in the office very agreeably to sign her part of the paperwork. But a few weeks later, when it was time to move some of her furniture into her new apartment, it was as if we were springing this awful change on her without warning, and with her increasing dementia, this is exactly what was happening in her mind. As we carried her dresser, some end tables, lamps and chairs outside to a friend's van, she screamed at us to stop stealing from her. No amount of patient explaining could sooth her impotent fury so she retreated upstairs and slammed her bedroom door.

Normally a very empathetic person, I could not allow myself to fully feel her sense of betrayal and pain or I would have been immobilized. It would have been too dangerous to let her stay at home alone and she was equally adamant about not moving in with us or having an aide move in with her. There was no solution that would please her.

Because Mark was the only one she trusted at this time, he stayed behind to try to comfort her while Bruce and I, with the help of our friend, brought the furniture over to Rose Hall and set up her apartment.

With trepidation, I called my mother the next morning to let her know what time we would be over to pick her up. I fully expected her either not to remember this was moving day or else to hang up on me in anger. Instead, she was surprisingly cheerful. I told her I'd bring a suitcase and help her pack whatever clothes she wanted to bring and she called me "an angel," a completely uncharacteristic expression. I was relieved, but wary, knowing her mood could change several more times before the day was over.

I don't know what was going on in my mother's mind that day, but I'm guessing she thought we were all going on vacation together. Up in her bedroom, with my suitcase spread out on her bed, we went through her dresses, picking out her favorites, along with jewelry to go with each one. She selected nightgowns, a robe, slippers, underwear, stockings, and shoes. The day before, I had selected some photographs, decorative objects and some of her favorite books so they would be in her new apartment when she arrived.

Arrival at Rose Hall went smoothly. After Bruce and I helped her unpack and arrange things where she wanted them, Dana, Jay and Mark joined us for a family dinner in a separate dining room at the assisted living facility, with my mother sitting happily at the head of the table. The whole day had gone much better than I had dared to hope for – until it was time for us to leave.

"Where are you going?" she demanded as we stood and began to put our coats on. "You can't leave me here alone! I thought we were all staying here." Her duplicitous family had tricked her and now they were sneaking out the door leaving her here with total strangers. She was still yelling at us as an aide gently guided her toward the elevator and we all guiltily made our way toward the door.

The next day, I left work early and stopped over at Rose Hall to see how she was doing. She was in the dining room sitting with another new resident at a table for four, gamely trying to carry on a conversation. The staff invited me to join her, so after a quick call to Bruce, I sat down for dinner and did my best to encourage this burgeoning friendship. Sometimes, I would take a break during the day and spontaneously check on her, hoping this would make her feel less abandoned and also let the staff know she was being watched out for by family. Too often, I found her sitting by herself in the dining room while the other residents chatted over meals, and I never saw her playing Bingo or cards with the other people.

When she was younger, she didn't warm quickly to new people. In addition to being shy, my mother had certain standards of dress and behavior that she expected people to follow, carried over from a more old-fashioned time when men wore jackets and ties and women wore dresses every day, not just for weddings and funerals. Poor grammar or vulgar language were not tolerated when my brother and I were children, and by the time I turned twelve, I was no longer allowed to wear shorts because they weren't ladylike. My mother always wore dresses and stockings, even when cleaning the house or doing something messy like painting the basement stairs. As an elderly woman, she dressed well, but not fashionably by contemporary standards.

So when I found her sitting by herself most of the time, instead of socializing with the other women, I thought she was looking down on them all for wearing slacks and, heaven forbid, sneakers. But then I noticed the same groups of people sitting together day after day in little cliques – the ones who still could remember how to play bridge or mahjong. The Bingo players and the arts and crafters all had their little circle of friends. It occurred to me that a new image might be swimming in her consciousness, something like a scene from Jane Austin where the ladies from the old, established gentry were sitting around the parlor playing whist and whispering about the obvious misfit who dared to think her presence would be tolerated among them. And my mother, dressed in her best blue dress and coordinating accessories, would instantly feel their disdain – why they could tell just by looking at her that she couldn't play their games – and she would retreat back upstairs to her strange hotel room and curse her wretched family for abandoning her like this.

Time and again, when I came to visit, I'd find her alone in her apartment and she'd lash out in anger at me for putting her in "this hell hole." That was a favorite expression now that she used repeatedly.

I tried very hard to be patient knowing she was going through a difficult adjustment, but one evening after work, I was tired and I lost my temper. "Do you know what a hell hole is," I asked with barely controlled rage. Her eyes grew wide and her mouth settled into a stern look of disapproval at my impertinence. "A hell hole is a room in a rat-infested slum with drug dealers and prostitutes doing business just outside your door so you'd be constantly afraid to ever leave your apartment. I'm tired of being yelled at for trying to do what's best for you. I know it hasn't been easy, but it's necessary!" And I left, letting the door slam behind me.

The next day when I came to see her, she was pleasant and I never heard her talk about her new home being a hellhole again. That surprised me because on so many other occasions, her memory seemed to be wiped clean of any recent events causing me to fear that our hellhole conversation was destined to be repeated over and over for the next several months. She and I had crossed over into a new dynamic.

2

When I was a child, she had suffered from depression and severe mood swings that made my brother and me tread very carefully around her lest we trigger an angry tirade. Life hadn't been easy for her ever since my father Arthur Christensen died in 1947 from complications after surgery to help relieve his emphysema and the lingering effects of a recent bout of pneumonia three months earlier. In September, my father had gone out to Montana to finish recuperating while visiting his parents. My brother was five and I was eighteen months old at the time which probably explains why our mother stayed back in Metuchen with us rather than accompanying him out west. While in Montana, he was diagnosed with a brain abscess and was rushed to the hospital in Anaconda. My mother flew out to be with him, but he died ten days later.

Then, just six months afterwards, while Mark was at kindergarten and my mother was putting my father's clothes away in the attic, I was playing alone in the living room. That was in the days before parents were warned to baby-proof every square inch of their homes with outlet plugs and gates blocking the stairs and locks on all the kitchen cabinets. I shudder to remember all the poisonous cleaning products under the sink and the unlabeled bottle of turpentine in the garage. The overhead pipes in the basement where Mark and I often played were covered with aging asbestos. So it's not surprising that my mother didn't look upon the heavy upholstered rocking chair that my brother and I loved to stand in while rocking furiously as anything but a benign piece of furniture. I can only imagine the horror and guilt she felt when she heard my screams of pain and found me pinned under the rocking chair with my face pressed against the exposed and very hot radiator.

Thankfully, I don't remember that day, but I can still see in my mind's eye a brightly lit hospital room and strangers dressed in white moving about me. There were many trips to the hospital over the next few years for plastic surgery, adding greatly to my mother's financial worries. The burden and loneliness of being widowed at 37 and raising two small children without any extended family nearby to help took a heavy toll on our family.

She found comfort in a glass of wine in the evening while escaping into the world of fiction found in her ever-changing pile of library books. In time, one glass wasn't enough to blur the anxiety and she began to buy her wine in gallon jugs.

~

On weekends, I would take my mother out for walks in Echo Lake Park in Mountainside or the park in the center of Westfield where, many years before, Bruce and I had posed for wedding photos. Usually, she liked escaping Rose Hall for a few hours with me, but on one occasion, she didn't want to leave. "I can't go with you," she explained with considerable agitation. "My husband is coming for me and I have to pack…. Where is my suitcase?"

Her bureau drawers were open, but she seemed confused about what she wanted to bring with her. A few things were piled on her bed with no apparent sense or order to them. Was she having some sort of premonition about her death or, more likely, was her mind back in the distant past when she was a young wife with a husband to look after her?

~

My father had been a research engineer specializing in metallurgy for the Anaconda Copper Company in Montana. He was born on May 22, 1905 in the village of Tordenskjold, Otter Tail County, Minnesota. His family lived for a few years in the small town of Underwood, Minnesota, before moving to Missoula, Montana when he was twelve. My grandfather Carl Christensen, who I never met and know very little about, had been a farmer back in Minnesota. By the time they were settled in Montana, he had become a union organizer during the tumultuous years of the growing labor movement in America. I know even less about my grandmother Martha Larson Christensen. They were both born in Minnesota to Danish and Norwegian immigrant farmers who chose Minnesota for its similarity to their native climate. Through Ancestry.com I met a distant Larson cousin who lives in Alberta, Canada. His research shows that the Larsons who came to America were descended from Lars Boe, a tenant farmer from the little town of Voss, Norway, not far from the city of Bergen.

According to my mother's older sister Mollie, my grandfather Carl was a radical socialist who was often out of work as a result of his strong union beliefs, and his family felt the financial hardship. My father had put himself through college and then helped his younger brothers Carlton and Chester get an education. With the prevailing attitude toward education for women, his younger sisters Bernice and Muriel probably never had a chance to go to college.

My mother had met her Montana in-laws only a few times and I got the impression from comments she made that, had they been next door neighbors, she wouldn't have gone out of her way to be more than just casual friends. She found their Scandinavian reticence strangely off-putting and I'm guessing they thought she was too citified and sophisticated. My mother said Muriel was married to a bad-tempered man named Charles who worked as a draftsman in Missoula. Census data show that he and Muriel were married by a justice of the peace in January of 1944 with no relatives as witnesses, which suggests they got married in a hurry because either he was about to go off to war or Muriel was pregnant. Charles seemed to feel it was his right to hit her even when his father-in-law was visiting. On one occasion, my grandfather sat quietly in the living room, minding his own business as he thought he should while his son-in-law and Muriel argued in the kitchen. He could hear his daughter scream as her husband hit her repeatedly and yet, apparently, he didn't think he had the right to intervene to protect her so he kept his emotions under tight control and went home and had a heart attack, non-fatal fortunately, but one can only wonder what would have happened if he had dared to speak up.

By the time my parents had met, my mother was working at the new Women's Clinic at New York Hospital and living in a small apartment in a Greenwich Village brownstone on 12th Street, and my father was working for the Raritan Copper Works in Perth Amboy, New Jersey. He lived in a rented room in a pretty house on Water Street, across from the Raritan Yacht Club. Most of the people they knew were involved in one way or another with the Anaconda Copper Company, and mutual friends introduced them in 1936.

My mother loved the excitement of New York City and all that it offered. She spoke of those years with great fondness because, even though many people were poor during the Great Depression, prices were cheap and she could still see a Broadway show or attend the opera with a standing room ticket, eat regularly and pay her rent – all on $12 a week. She was proud of being self-sufficient in the rough world of Depression-era New York.

In her twenties, my mother was a red-haired, blue-eyed beauty with a striking resemblance to a young Grace Kelly. My father was tall and dark-haired with the slender build of a Fred Astaire. Back in Montana, my father had lived and worked in Anaconda, the town next to Butte, which was twenty miles away, but they didn't meet until they had both traveled more than 2,000 miles from home.

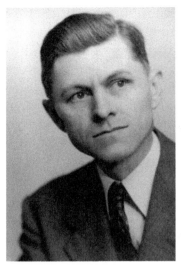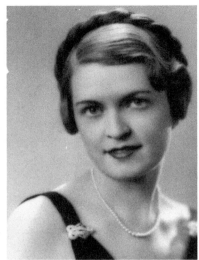

My parents, Arthur Christensen and Eileen O'Meara, met in New York in 1936 and married the following year. (Photos by Amé Dupont, New York)

During their courtship, my father took my mother dancing and to the theater or to parties at the Laist's elegant house in Scarsdale or their apartment on Fifth Avenue. Fred and Rosalba Laist were like surrogate parents to my mother when she came to New York at the age of twenty. Uncle Fred was a senior Vice President in the Anaconda Company's New York office with several successful patents bringing in a healthy income. He and Rosalba knew my mother's family back in Butte and offered to keep an eye on her when she moved east. They had three grown children around my mother's age so she was included in weekend house parties and other family gatherings where she was thrown in with the privileged few who were safe from the harsh realities of unemployment and poverty. As a young, impressionable woman she listened to the disdainful criticism of Franklin Roosevelt's Works Progress Administration and his Civilian Conservation Corp. These wealthy people didn't approve of anything Roosevelt did to put people to work and get money back into circulation, but she loved and respected the Laists so she registered as a Republican and dutifully voted in every election. She was too young when her parents died to have known her father was a dedicated Democrat who would probably have been appalled at her lack of loyalty to the party of the working people. Even her grandfather Marco Medin, a millionaire entrepreneur, had progressive values that would later be more closely identified with the Democratic Party as it existed in the 1930's.

As an up-and-coming young engineer with Anaconda, my father fit in well with the Laists and their circle of friends. In reaction to the financial hardship caused by his father's ardent union organizing, I suspect my father leaned in the opposite direction and aligned himself with management.

Because my mother and I would always end up crying whenever I asked her questions about him, I wrote to my Aunt Mollie out in Butte and asked her to tell me everything she knew about my father. She recounted an incident at the copper smelter in Anaconda, Montana, where my father worked before he was sent east. Mining and smelting were hard, dangerous work and many violent disputes broke out between labor and management. Numerous strikes on behalf of labor broke out for better wages and safer working conditions while management tried to break the unions by bringing in non-union workers and armed security guards to protect the mines and smelters. Because my father was a college-educated engineer, he was expected to join with management in a lock-out of the Anaconda smelter. Whether he did this under duress to keep his job during the Depression or because of a genuine loyalty to the company, it caused a rift between my father and grandfather that I suspect lasted for the rest of their lives.

After my father died and I was seriously burned, my mother wrote to his family back in Montana. I don't know if she might have been hoping they could help with my medical bills, but Carlton's terse reply let her know that, while they sympathized with her problems, she should not expect anything from them. Mark and I never even got birthday cards from our Christensen relatives. Since I had never met them, their indifference didn't really bother me as a child, and Mom had wisely arranged for surrogate grandparents in the form of "Aunt" Carrie and "Uncle" Mac, my elderly godparents who did an admirable job of filling the void on holidays and birthdays. It was only many years later, when I was a parent myself, that I began to be curious about grandparents and siblings who could behave as though their son's and brother's children didn't exist.

When I began doing family research on Ancestry.com, I found a link to a site that shows photographs of graves in cemeteries all over the country. Right there in the Missoula City Cemetery, I found a photo of my Christensen grandparents' tombstone showing that Carl died in 1952, and Martha died in 1947. It appeared that my grandmother had died the same year as my father so I thought, "No wonder we never heard from her!" How could I be angry with her? If she hadn't died prematurely, I was sure she would have loved us.

In 2015, Bruce and I went to Missoula so I could see where my father had grown up, but sadly, Interstate 90 had cut through town in the 1960's and obliterated his house, the address of which I had found through old Census records. I got out of the car anyway and took pictures of the grassy hillside at the edge of the highway where his house had once stood. Then, we went to the cemetery and searched up and down the rows of headstones looking for my grandparents' final resting place. It was a huge cemetery, and after looking in vain for some time, Bruce found a cemetery GPS app on his phone that led us right to Carl and Martha whose tombstone clearly revealed, in better light, that she had died in 1974, not 1947. I was livid and my eyes stung with tears as I realized my grandmother had lived to be 90 and never once in all those years did she care enough to reach out to Mark and me.

When we got home, I dug out my parents' old photo album from the late 1930's. In 1938, they had gone back to Montana for Ginny Laist's wedding which was held at her parents' huge log cabin "mansion" on Georgetown Lake. While they were out there, they went to Missoula to visit his family and, of course, pictures were taken. My father is shown standing happily among these people whom he hadn't seen in several years and there in the group are a stern-looking man and woman who appear to be in their mid- fifties so I am guessing they must be my father's parents Martha and Carl. No one thought to label the photos, unfortunately, but the same woman and man are also in a picture of Amon B. Larson's tombstone, taken during a visit back to Dalton, Minnesota. Amon was Martha's father who was born in Norway in 1836. (Amon came here at the age of 21 in 1857 and within a few years was fighting in the Civil War as a private in Wisconsin's 20th Regiment. Amon married Britta Mikkelsdotter and Martha was the youngest of their six children.)

It's entirely appropriate that Martha and Carl would look somber standing in a cemetery, but another photo showed them posing with a little girl about 4 years old, probably their first grandchild, and a newborn infant in the arms of either their daughter Bernice or Muriel. By the late 1930's people *did* smile in photographs, especially when standing with their precious grandchildren, but not Martha and Carl. These were cold looking people.

When I was a child, I would sometimes wonder which would hurt more – losing my father when I was ten or twelve years old or losing him when I was too young to realize what happened. Since I was only eighteen months old when he died, I have no recollection of him now. But at the age of three, I must have still had some lingering memories of him and wondered where he was. I clearly remember sitting on the walkway by the back porch on a warm summer day, watering the rhubarb with my toy watering can. A wasp landed on the walk next to me, and in the innocent logic of a three-year-old, I thought it would be appropriate to pour water on the wasp, too. The wasp responded by stinging me in the delicate skin between two fingers on my left hand. It's amazing to me now how vividly I still remember crying for my mother who rushed out the back door to see what was wrong. She scooped me up in her arms, tended as best she could to the pain, and then cuddled me in the rocking chair as she crooned, "Bye Baby Bunting, Daddy's gone a hunting to catch a brand new rabbit's skin to wrap my Baby Bunting in." I remember thinking, as clearly as if it were a few days ago, "So that's where he went!"

Being four years older, Mark had very strong memories of happy times curled up in our father's lap listening to stories or watching him create toys out of pieces of wood left over from his more serious projects. I would ask Mark questions about what life was like in our house before our father died, but a five-year-old has a very limited frame of reference. It didn't take long for me to conclude as a child that, if my father had to die, I would have preferred being old enough to have had some lasting memories and a sense that I really knew him even though it would have meant having to go through the grieving process that I had been spared as a baby.

Many years later, while cleaning out my mother's house, I came across a handwritten draft of a 1940's letter my father had written to his congressman asking him not to support joining the conflict in Europe. I was amazed to learn he was an isolationist, not apparently concerned about the Nazi atrocities until I realized later that he was looking at the latest turmoil in Europe from the perspective of someone who had grown up during the "Great War to end all wars" and was naturally skeptical about the necessity for the US to get involved in yet another European conflict. Perhaps at the time he wrote his letter, he didn't know much about the full horror of what the Nazis were doing. Isolationism was the prevailing mood of the country prior to the Japanese attack on Pearl Harbor. Once we were attacked on December 7, 1941, even my pregnant mother was so enraged, she said she wished she could enlist and go fight the Japanese.

With war came an urgent need for more copper that was used in the manufacture of munitions and wire for expanded communications. Because my father was working on improving methods for extracting usable copper from the low-grade ore that was once discarded, his job was considered essential for the war effort and he received a draft deferment. He didn't get sent overseas, but he did spend long periods of time away from home working at various copper mining locations and refineries out west. And when he was back in New Jersey, he spent long hours working overtime at the smelter in Perth Amboy.

It could have been a lonely time for my mother, but she had my infant brother to keep her busy, a Victory garden of vegetables to tend and the new challenge of keeping house under the rationing system. The Office of Civilian Defense called upon each American family to become a "fighting unit on the home front," so my mother dutifully recycled toothpaste tubes, string, aluminum foil scraps, tin cans, newspapers and, on the rare occasions when she had enough ration coupons to buy bacon, she'd pour the fat into a can and take that to the salvage people because fats were used to make glycerin which was essential for making explosives. A newsreel at the time reported that enough glycerin to make ten billion rapid-fire cannon shells was thrown out each year so housewives were exhorted to regard their skillets of bacon fat as little munitions factories and save every drop. She took her patriotic duty to ration scarce resources for the good of the troops very seriously so when a neighbor bragged that her family thought rationing was silly and bought all the coffee, butter, meat, cigarettes and stockings they wanted on the black market, Mom had nothing but contempt for her, even long after the war was over.

As World War II was coming to a close in the summer of 1945, my parents decided it was safe to have another child and I was conceived that July, putting me in the front of the huge post war baby boom generation of children born to returning service men who had put their lives on hold for four long years and were eager to get caught up. I was born in April of 1946 at a time when giving birth seemed to call for solicitous pampering of new mothers. It was a normal delivery and yet my mother was kept in the hospital to recuperate for two weeks. When she came home, my father hired a baby nurse to take care of me and do the cooking and cleaning for six weeks, a luxury few women enjoy today.

But only a few months after my birth, my father began losing weight and suffered from a chronic, debilitating cough. He was diagnosed with emphysema, brought on by heavy smoking and working in the foul environment of a copper smelter.

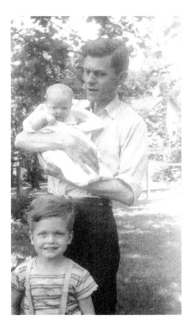

A faded photograph from that time shows my painfully thin father holding me at the age of 4 or 5 months while my four-year-old brother smiled at the camera. Judging from their wedding photographs, my vibrant, productive father had always been slender, but by this time, he looked almost skeletal. My mother now had an infant, a preschooler and an invalid to care for.

3

Right after my father died, Aunt Mollie urged my mother to sell our house in Metuchen and use the money to go on a long cruise for the purpose of finding a new husband, preferably a very rich one. My mother chose the more practical route of keeping the house that meant security to Mark and me and renting out the spare bedrooms to a succession of Rutgers graduate students and local high school teachers. The finished attic bedroom, with its own private bath, was rented to Mr. Hitchcock, a middle-aged Englishman with a red sports car he whimsically named Josephine.

My mother hated having strangers in the house, but there were few options available to widows with young children in those days. There were no day care centers back then and whatever she would have been able to earn as a secretary would have been taken up completely with babysitting expenses. She was determined to preserve my father's life insurance money as protection for Mark and me in case anything happened to her.

But as much as my mother hated renting rooms to strangers, my brother and I thought it was fun having different young men, like a succession of uncles, visiting for a few months at a time, especially the Rutgers graduate students who would play with us, and even my mother appreciated the extra help when it was time to take down the screens and put up the storm windows or mount the last of the kitchen cabinets my father had been building before he got sick. Mr. Hitchcock gave Mark and me gifts at Christmas, and that, combined with the fact that he'd been living in the attic for as long as I could remember, and he occasionally gave us rides in Josephine, made him seem almost like family. When I was four or five years old, he even took all of us down to the Jersey shore for the day, the first time Mark and I had ever seen the ocean. Josephine wasn't big enough to accommodate all four of us so he must have driven my father's 1940 Desoto that my mother had recently learned how to drive.

As soon as I started first grade, everything changed. My mother got a job in a local doctor's office, the "roomers" had to find new living arrangements, and I got my own room back with pink walls, ruffled curtains and stuffed animals on the bed. Being four years older, Mark was supposed to walk me to school and wait for me after school for the walk back, but four years was too big a gap for us to be friends and not quite big enough for him to feel protective of me. As a result, we squabbled all the way to school with him unable to resist his need to tease me and me unable to muster the necessary will power to ignore him. After I repeatedly threw my lunch box at him, breaking a substantial number of glass thermos bottles, I was allowed to walk the mile or so to school by myself or with friends. I was also entrusted with my own house key, fastened inside my coat pocket with a big diaper pin, but I wasn't allowed to go out and play after school until I had called my mother at work so she'd know I had made it home safely.

In the early 1950's, before every family in the neighborhood had a television, we kids played outside until dark or until our stinging toes drove us inside to warm up for a while. The houses on our end of Clarendon Court were built between 1910 and 1920, but a little beyond our house, the paved road ended in a wild expanse of woods with a pond for skating, a steep, winding hill for sledding, a deep ravine covered in vines that, in our vivid imaginations, looked like a dungeon, and an authentically scary "Dead Man's Cave," where a workman had been killed when a pedestrian tunnel collapsed under the Pennsylvania Railroad tracks. Since the main line of the Pennsylvania Railroad ran alongside the woods, occasional hobo sightings added to our sense of daring adventure. As long as I called my mother after school to let her know I had arrived safely and rushed home at the sound of the five o'clock whistle to put the potatoes in the oven, I was free to do whatever I pleased in between and felt lucky not to have a mother who hovered.

During the day, she worked at a responsible job, then came home around 6:00 p.m. and started dinner. If the day had been especially stressful or something else had triggered a bad mood, she'd pour herself a glass of wine right away and dinner would often end up overdone. Mark and I knew better than to be finicky eaters so we ate whatever was put before us. But on Sundays, my mother enjoyed preparing meals that made up for the rest of the week. Her mashed potatoes were the best I've ever had anywhere and the memory of her roast pork with crisp, oven-roasted potatoes can still make my mouth water. Another favorite was chicken fried in bacon fat, producing an enticingly fragrant aroma that wafted out over the neighborhood on warm summer evenings, drawing Mark and me inside for dinner with genuine enthusiasm. Despite her Irish heritage, she never served corned beef and cabbage or Irish soda bread, even on St. Patrick's Day. The Irish were never known for their cuisine so we ate classic "American" food, like steak and roast beef or turkey with real home-made gravy, not the kind from a jar.

We ate most of our meals in the breakfast nook my father had built out of the former pantry. He had been in the middle of modernizing the kitchen and building new dining room furniture when he got sick. He had also loved to paint landscapes in oil, build toys for us and design the modern dream house he planned to build one day. Down in the basement, he had a fully-equipped work area and an assortment of power tools needed for his various projects.

My mother had once said my father would have made a perfectly happy hermit because, when he got home from work, or on weekends, he was content to pursue his many interests, all of which could be done alone. When they were first married, she had wanted to continue working but, in those days when jobs were scarce, it was considered selfish for a woman to work when she had a husband to support her so she dutifully stayed home to keep house. She did her best to master the housewifely skills of cooking, cleaning and decorating, but a three-room apartment occupied by two people didn't require her full attention for eight hours a day so she spent much of her time escaping into the much more interesting world of books. Ever since she was a young child of four or five, when she taught herself how to unlock the mystery of letters on a page, she had retreated to a quiet corner to escape.

Years later, as a young widow with two children, she kept a stack of magazines and library books by her place at the kitchen table so she could escape into a less stressful world while we ate. Mark soon followed her example and read his comic books while I looked at the cartoons and story illustrations in the *Saturday Evening Post*. It would be a few years before I could read, so I passed the time trying to guess what the words under the pictures meant. As long as we didn't make too much noise and distract our mother from her books, Mark and I were allowed to let our hamsters run around on the dinner table and help themselves to vegetables, something we smugly knew our friends' mothers would have found appalling. She was often tired and cranky, but watching a hamster try to jam an entire string bean into its overstuffed pouch could still make her laugh.

4

We had moved my mother into assisted living a few weeks before Christmas 1998. By late January, she had come down with the flu and a cough so severe I was afraid she had pneumonia so I left work early and took her to the doctor. The X-rays indicated nothing more than bronchitis, but a complete physical a few weeks later revealed a large growth on one of her ovaries.

In a case of perverse irony, I came down with an even worse case of the flu and on the day I was supposed to take her to Overlook Hospital for additional tests, I was running a fever of 104 and was admitted to the hospital with bilateral, atypical pneumonia. Over the ten day period I was hospitalized, 28 people had died from pneumonia and the doctors weren't sure at one point if I would survive because atypical pneumonia doesn't respond to antibiotics.

I wasn't worried about getting better until a minister started paying me visits every day to solemnly pray over me. If I died from pneumonia, it would seem like some cruel curse had been visited upon our family. And my poor mother, sitting alone in her strange hotel room, would wonder what had happened to me. If someone explained to her that pneumonia had killed me, would she remember that awful day in October 1918 when she came down the stairs for the first time after recovering

from the Spanish Flu to find three coffins in the living
room?

~

My mother was the youngest of eight children in a
devoutly Irish Catholic family.

She was born in 1910, to Sarah Medin and John J.
O'Meara. He was an Irish immigrant who came to this
country from Bunmahon in 1880 at the age of 15 to work
as a pit boy in the copper mines of Butte, Montana. His
mother was Anastasia Harney who was born in County
Waterford in 1821, in Stradbally-Ballylaneen Parish. Her
first husband was John Patrick Kane, originally spelled
Keane, and they had six children, the last of whom was
also named John Patrick. He had an older brother whose
first name was Patrick, as well a sister named Honora,
and three more brothers named William, Richard and
Edward.

When her first husband died in 1857 when he was
only 47, Anastasia married John Joseph O'Meara and,
at the age of 44, she gave birth to their first child, my
grandfather, who was also named John Joseph. Three
years later, their son Michael was born. When I look at
the genealogical chart, my head swims with all the Johns,
Patricks, Richards and Michaels. Most of the women were
named Sarah, Mary, Honora and Anastasia.

I had always thought my grandfather came from the
city of Waterford, but actually Irish people often identify
with their home county rather than the small town where
they lived. It wasn't until 2005 when Dana gave me *Last
of the Donkey Pilgrims* that I put the pieces together and
realized Bunmahon is where he was born. The author,

Kevin O'Hara, spent about a year traveling around the ring of Ireland walking beside a tinker's cart pulled by a lovable donkey named Missie. (Out of consideration for Missie, he didn't ride on the cart as most tinkers did.) On his journey, he met dozens of rural Irish families who gave him a meal and a bed for the night and a field where Missie could graze, and in exchange, he would entertain them with his stories.

It was when he passed through the tiny village of Bunmahon on the southern coast of Ireland that he learned about Ireland's copper mines that had become less profitable once cheaper Cuban copper became available, about the same time that copper, silver and gold were discovered in Butte, Montana, so half the town had emigrated to Butte. But at least the town was fairly well off during the famine years and was able to help many struggling people in the hard-hit counties. After reading O'Hara's account of his visit to the village, I dug out the old family Bible and found an overlooked reference to Bunmahon squeezed into the space between my grandfather's name and County Waterford.

In September of 2006, Bruce and I visited Ireland for the first time. I especially wanted to see Bunmahon as we traveled the coast road from Dublin to Shannon during our all-too-brief stay. As we descended the hill into Bunmahon from Tankardstown, my excitement grew. We parked in front of a pub but found, to our surprise, that it was closed. So was the fish and chip shop next door. Not really expecting to find any relatives still living in town, I thought I would have to be content with collecting some shells and pebbles from the beach and taking pictures of any buildings old enough to have been there when my grandfather was a boy. The village seemed strangely deserted except for one woman on the beach who, in response to a query from Bruce, said she thought there was still an O'Meara family in town and suggested we go asking door-to-door.

As we walked up the one main street through town, a black lab sleeping in the road perked up when he saw what might be the only activity in town that day. Then a pug, barking at us from behind a low wall, jumped over and the two dogs accompanied us as we went door-to-door looking for any relatives who might still live there. At the third house, a woman said there was a Michael O'Meara living in a house called Sea Spray and she pointed toward the upper coast road.

We found the house, built close to the road with a low wall around it and painted the traditional mustard yellow. When a dark-haired man with glasses came to the door, I said, "I'm looking for Michael O'Meara."

"Well, that would be me!" he said in a heavy Irish brogue.

"My grandfather John J. O'Meara left Bunmahon in 1880 at the age of 15 to go work in the copper mines of Butte, Montana," I replied, hoping this little bit of information was something he had heard before.

"Come in! Come in!" he exclaimed and called his mother Peggie who had been napping in the bedroom. They put the tea kettle on and we spent the rest of the day comparing stories we had heard about our families. Michael and Peggie's brogues were so thick, I had to sit on the edge of my chair and strain to understand what they were saying making me wonder if our American accents were equally difficult for them. It turned out Michael's grandfather, also named Michael, was my grandfather's younger brother. Peggie was married to my mother's first cousin John who had died in 2004. (As far as I know, my mother never knew about her Irish cousins.)

The O'Meara family, including Michael's wife Ann and their two children Mairead and Sean, are still living in our great grandparents' house overlooking the Irish Sea with rolling pastures sloping down to a cliff walk. Anastasia and John rented the tiny house and small kitchen garden from an English physician named George Walker, since in those days most land was still owned by absentee landlords and the Irish had few rights. The house still had a thatched roof up until the 1940's, and in the kitchen, the outline of the big fireplace where Anastasia cooked the family meals is still visible, although now cabinets fill the space and additional rooms have been added on to the traditional one-room cottage. Michael's grandfather had briefly gone to Butte to work in the mines but returned home to help his aging parents on the farm.

I had planned to visit the local church cemetery to search for my great-grandparents' gravesites, but Michael assured me we would never find the cemetery on our own. We were glad we had accepted his offer to show us the way because we truly would not have been able to navigate the winding, narrow roads, some not much wider than cow paths, that led to Faugheen Cemetery at the site of an ancient Cistercian monastery in the middle of lush cattle pastures. A tiny white chapel, big enough to hold 25 people at most, sits in front of the cemetery. On the day we were there, the air was filled with the scent of freshly-mown hay from the surrounding farms and cattle were grazing on the adjacent fields.

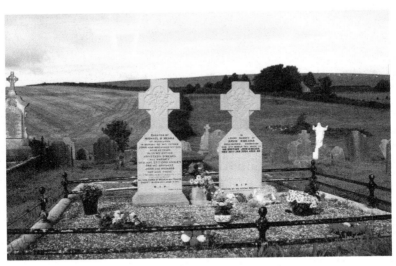

I walked around the family gravesite and found an inscription that suddenly brought tears to my eyes. (Photo taken by the author)

John and Anastasia O'Meara's gravesite is marked by a beautiful Celtic cross with a black wrought iron railing around the family plot. I walked around the gravesite and found an inscription that suddenly brought tears to my eyes, *"This railing was erected by John J. O'Meara of Butte, Montana, USA, in memory of his parents."* It must have pained him greatly that he had lived apart from his family for most of his life and that he was so far away when his parents died. In all the years he was living and working in Montana, he had sent money home to his parents, helping them to buy the house and farm and live a more comfortable life, but in the end, all he could do was pay for a railing to honor their memory. I had never realized until this visit how much being connected to these people I had never met would mean to me.

Before continuing on our trip the following day, we stopped back at the house for one last visit and, of course, a cup of tea. When it was time to leave, we exchanged hugs and, as we headed toward the front door, Peggie said in her lilting brogue, "Ah no, not that way. Use the back door; you're family!" I'll always treasure those words.

Cousin Michael and his wife built two vacation cottages on the family farm to supplement their income from raising cattle. In 2010, we returned to Ireland, this time with Dana and Carlos and Jay and Deané, and rented the cottage that overlooks the cattle pasture with the Irish Sea in the distance. Michael's friend Jim spent a day with us sharing his knowledge of Bunmahon's history and giving us a tour of the Geo Park and the Copper Coast Heritage Center.

One day, Michael took Bruce and me on a cliff walk behind his cattle pasture. We had to climb over stone walls, under electrified fences, up rocky ravines and through herds of cattle, including past one very suspicious bull, but it was worth it. The views behind the O'Meara's pastures rival anything we saw at the Cliffs of Moher or the Ring of Kerry. The cliff walk along the Copper Coast is one of Ireland's best kept secrets and I think the people of Bunmahon want to keep it that way.

As we were walking, I kept thinking of my grandfather and his younger brother Michael playing in these fields and on the beach a short walk from their house, if indeed, they were even given time to play in those days when children were put to work early.

When I was growing up, I had heard the stories about my grandfather's older half brothers William, Patrick, Richard, Edward and John Patrick Kane who had emigrated to Butte in the 1870's to work in the copper mines. Of course, at that time, I didn't know they came from a long line of experienced miners or that most of their village emigrated at the same time. Because of their experience, some of the brothers worked their way up quickly and became mine superintendents. As soon as he was considered old enough to make the trip, my grandfather was sent to join his brothers, leaving probably from Cork or Cobh, known as Queenstown back then.

What a wrenching ordeal it must have been for my great-grandparents to send their children thousands of miles from home, not knowing when, or if, they would ever see them again. I remember how sad I felt when Dana went off to college even though I knew it would be a wonderful experience for her and we'd still be able to see her during visits throughout the school year. Cornell was only a four hours' drive away and we were so proud and happy for her when she was accepted at a school that would help open doors for her in a very competitive job market. The sadness was really caused by the realization that her childhood was over too soon and that after graduation, she might never come home to stay with us again. Their children's ability to be independent one day is what parents work toward from the very beginning and yet letting go is still heartbreaking.

I try to imagine what it must have been like for an unsophisticated country boy of 15, who had probably never been any further from home than the next village, to get on a sailing vessel, or maybe one of the first steam ships, and travel across the ocean to one of the big east coast cities like New York or Boston, then travel by train to Red Rock, the terminus of the Utah and Northern Railroad, and then finish the journey by stage coach through rugged mountain terrain all the way to Butte, straddling the Continental Divide. He didn't see his mother again until 1901 when he was married with several children of his own, and sadly, by then his father was already dead.

I have so many questions with no one in the family left to answer them. Did he travel with other young men he knew from Bunmahon or did he have to journey almost half way around the world entirely with strangers? Did his older brothers wire the money for his passage, using the new transcontinental and trans-Atlantic telegraph lines which must have seemed like magic to them, or did his parents scrape together just enough money to get him to Butte, causing more financial strain on the family? The former is more likely since the rapid expansion of international telegraph lines connecting the United States with Europe and the far East was the reason copper miners were in such great demand in Butte in the first place.

5

In 1891, my grandfather married Sarah Medin, the daughter of Marco Medin and Sarah Thornton. Marco was a Dalmatian count born May 4, 1824 in Budva, Montenegro, then the southernmost part of the Austrian Empire. Budva is a tiny medieval walled city on the Adriatic coast, a smaller and less grand version of Dubrovnik to the north.

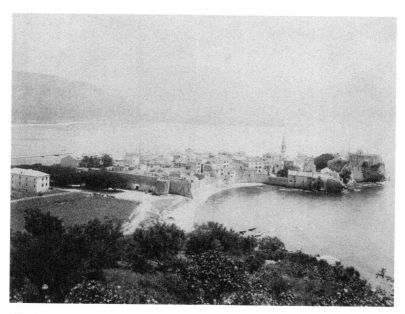

Budva is a tiny medieval walled city on the Adriatic coast, a smaller and less grand version of Dubrovnik to the north. (Photograph of Budva Bay by Franz Thiard de Laforest (Vienna, 1838 – Kotor, 1911)

He was the son of Anton Medin, a merchant from a prominent family, and Antonija Mikula. Anton and Antonija married young, had three sons and two daughters in quick succession, and then he died at the age of thirty-three. In her grief, Antonija gave a painting of the Madonna to their parish church in Anton's memory and attached a miniature locket that had been his. Marco's mother lived until 1896, but I don't know anything about her except that, according to Aunt Mollie, she was reputed to have been very haughty and overbearing to the servants which leads me to believe I wouldn't have liked her at all.

Family legend says that Marco's family pledged him in marriage to a young woman he adamantly did not want to marry. His grandmother felt so sorry for him being stuck in what would be a loveless marriage that she gave him enough money (Aunt Mollie said it was $50,000, but that would have been more than a million dollars back then) to leave Budva in the hope that his betrothed would grow tired of waiting for him and marry someone else. Since it was fashionable back then for wealthy young men to take the Grand Tour of Europe before settling down, his mother allowed him to set off with his tutor to visit the cultural meccas of the time, only according to Aunt Mollie, Marco ditched his tutor somewhere in Europe and jumped on a ship headed for America, leaving the poor young woman to retreat in sorrow and shame to a convent. At least, that was Aunt Mollie's version. Since Mollie was sixteen years older than my mother and spent many hours at her grandmother Sarah's side listening to stories about her adventurous life, she became our family historian by default.

Records at the National Archives show that Marco, accompanied by his brother Alexander who was 4 years younger, arrived in Philadelphia on the sailing ship *City of Glascow* on October 3, 1853. The ship, built in 1850, combined sails with steam power and took about 10 days to cross from Liverpool to Philadelphia.

Marco was 29 years old, a little older than I had expected, and his occupation was listed as "merchant." The family legend has them getting here soon after gold was discovered in California which must have excited their entrepreneurial spirit no end because they booked passage for a ship heading for Panama, crossed the isthmus and then picked up another ship heading north to San Francisco. It was probably more likely that they had heard of the Gold Rush while still in Europe and this is what drew them here in the first place. Aunt Mollie never mentioned Alexander, but later Census records show that he was here in the country.

I have no idea how much time all this traveling from Budva to San Francisco took and I wish we had letters or a diary recounting all the adventures they must have had and even the logistics of traveling before the age of credit cards, travelers checks or ATMs. I would love to have known the mental process by which Marco decided that going by sea would be preferable to the overland route since both methods of travel had their perils, but he certainly was not alone in taking the Panama route. I had thought at first that he was one of a small number of adventurers who dared to cross the hot, mosquito-infested jungles of Panama, risking yellow fever and malaria. I had envisioned him camping along the way and perhaps fighting off alligators and deadly snakes.

But the magic of the internet revealed an 1850's version of Trip Advisor for the thousands of people flocking to California in search of riches. Numerous hotels dotted the route and before booking a room, travelers could check the "complementary cards" signed by prior travelers who were happy with the accommodations. The steamships carrying passengers from many east coast and gulf ports to Panama or around Cape Horn were also rated and a person wishing to go to San Francisco, the most sought after destination, had many ships from which to choose. East coast newspapers posted lists of passengers leaving by ship for California on a daily basis.

Since the cost per person for passage by sea was considerably higher than for the overland route, it was usually only wealthier people who could choose to travel that way. But because so many people were eager to make the journey to California, ships were often overbooked, forcing passengers to sleep on deck or in tiered berths in crowded compartments. Once they got to the Atlantic side of the isthmus, people had to travel up the Charges River and then continue by mule through the jungle to the Pacific coast where they booked passage on a ship bound for San Francisco. By 1855, a railroad traversed the Isthmus of Panama, but when Marco and Alexander made the journey, it took about five days to cross, and the whole trip from New York to San Francisco was anywhere from four to eight weeks, depending upon weather conditions.

I can imagine the fascinating conversations that he and my great-grandmother Sarah Thornton had years later as they compared their journeys to the American west.

Sarah was an Irish immigrant born in Ballinrobe, County Mayo on December 15, 1839. She crossed the

Atlantic at about the age of six with her parents Anthony and Nancy Glyn Thornton and several siblings, taking six weeks to make the journey in a sailing vessel from Liverpool, England to New York City. They were among the fortunate few with the financial resources to escape Ireland during the terrible famine years when more than a million Irish people starved to death while their English landlords looked the other way.

Anthony, who had trained as a landscape designer in Germany, had been commissioned by a wealthy man to design the gardens on his estate outside Philadelphia. The position included a house for the growing Thornton family, and they stayed there for several years before moving to the suburb of Abington, Pennsylvania where her younger sister Maggie was born. It wasn't long before Anthony decided to join the land rush west of the Mississippi in the new state of Iowa. He bought a fertile tract of land in what became the town of Burlington and moved his family of ten children out there to settle.

At the age of sixteen, Sarah left her parents and younger sisters Maggie and Katie in Iowa and ventured across the Great Plains in a wagon train in 1855 with her older sister Annie and her husband Henry Garland. The other Thornton children were older and married, including Sarah's oldest sister Mary who had married a man with the last name of Dailey and had settled in California.

Annie had tuberculosis, and according to Aunt Mollie, Annie's doctor thought that living outdoors would be good for her health. Henry took this as an opportunity to sell his harness business and sign them up for an overland trip to California via wagon train, and Sarah came along to keep her sister company. Again, I wish these relatives had kept diaries because a rugged journey on rutted trails, across the desert, over treacherous rivers and mountains and through the lands inhabited by desperate and sometimes hostile Native Americans doesn't seem like good therapy for a potentially fatal illness. But in doing research for this family history, I found that the lure of free land and bountiful riches were not all that was promised by the promotional pamphlets and trail guides in circulation during the middle of the 19th Century. People were eager to believe that California's warm climate and lush vegetation would promote good health for everyone so that even if they never saw so much as an ounce of gold, this arduous journey to an idyllic land of milk and honey would be more than worth it.

Sarah, Henry and Annie probably started their trip near Council Bluffs, Iowa, one of several jumping off points along the Missouri River where emigrants could buy the wagons, oxen or mules and the many tools and other provisions that were needed for the long and difficult trip across the country.

In June of 2017, Bruce and I took a road trip from the Missouri River, heading west along the Platte River in Nebraska to Fort Kearny where the Oregon, California and Mormon Trails converged. Fort Kearny was established by the U.S. Government to provide assistance to the emigrants heading west, and it was the logical starting place for many of the wagon trains to assemble since the river valley provided an east-west highway along the flat prairie, as well as drinking water and plentiful grass for the oxen, horses or mules.

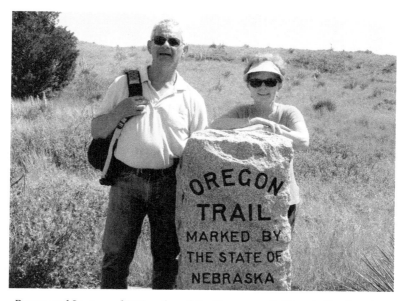

Bruce and I retraced 550 miles of the Oregon – California Trail trying to imagine what Great Grandma Sarah experienced in a wagon train in 1855. (Photo taken by anonymous hiker)

I am guessing that Sarah, Henry and Annie joined up with other emigrants at Fort Kearny for safety and the benefit of traveling with guides who had made the trip before. Aunt Mollie said they joined a caravan of 128 covered wagons, one of the largest wagon trains of the time, so the Indians chose not to bother them. However, many years later, Sarah entertained her grandchildren with stories about the smoldering wagons and massacred pioneers she passed on her journey west. This might have been a case of story-telling hyperbole because modern historians say the Indians got a bad rap. For the most part, the Indians that the pioneers encountered were very peaceful and liked trading with the people heading out west. They also served as guides and many emigrant journals written at the time tell about friendly meetings where goods were traded and meals were shared among white and Indian families. The Sioux, Shoshone and Paiute guided thousands of emigrants through their tribal territories and it wasn't until a bit later, when the settlers began to overwhelm the grasslands, kill off the buffalo just for sport, and repeatedly violate treaties that were intended to protect the Indian's homelands that hostile encounters became more common. I suspect that exaggerated stories about Indian atrocities were simply a way to justify the horrible mistreatment the Indians suffered at the hands of white settlers and the U.S. Government.

As Bruce and I drove along route 26 in Nebraska, which runs parallel to the Platte River, I tried to imagine what it must have been like traveling by wagon train in 1855. Emigrants started out in late April or May when the grass on the prairie was plentiful enough to provide food for the draft animals, as well as the small herds of cattle and goats that many pioneers brought with them for meat and milk on the journey. With all the overland traffic, it didn't take long for the grass to get worn down and clouds of dust to fill the air, choking travelers and animals alike. For that reason, the wagons didn't follow each other single file as artists' renderings often show, but rather spread out in a wide path as each family tried to avoid "eating dust."

As far as the eye can see the Nebraska prairie seems monotonously flat for hundreds of miles, but upon closer view, there are thousands of gullies and dry stream beds around which the wagon trains had to navigate. Rivers were a much more difficult challenge. If they were lucky, the emigrants were able to cross rivers where enterprising settlers or local Indians were willing to ferry the wagons across for about $4 per wagon. A large wagon train, like the one Sarah traveled in, probably took several days to get everyone across. The Platte, which means flat in French, was an unusual river in that it was very wide and shallow in most places. Emigrants described it as "a mile wide and a foot deep," but there were dangerous places where, after a heavy rain, the water was suddenly much deeper, causing panic among the draft animals, sometimes leading to capsized wagons and tragic drownings. In other places, the Platte River bottom turned to quicksand with equally tragic consequences.

I had read about the formidable Platte River and seen artists' renderings showing hundreds of wagons lined up to cross the wide expanse so I was surprised to see how small it is today. When Bruce and I were on the top of Scotts Bluff in western Nebraska looking out over the river and surrounding prairie, we met a man who had grown up in the area. He told us the river has been dammed in several locations along its route in order to create reservoirs for crop irrigation. As a result, the Platte is a meandering stream compared with its former size.

Bruce did almost all the driving which was an arrangement that seemed to please us both. He's more comfortable behind the wheel rather than being a passenger, and I was happily free to transport myself back in time so I could imagine what Sarah was experiencing. Of course, riding in an air-conditioned car on a paved highway is nothing like what the early emigrants experienced. But I could appreciate the enormity of the great plains that seem to go on forever in all directions. Thankfully, there were no billboards on the route we traveled and the landscape was broken only occasionally by silos or barns off in the distance, so I could understand the eager anticipation the emigrants felt when they knew from their guide books that it was time to be on the lookout for several of the awe-inspiring landmarks that previous pioneers had written about with great enthusiasm.

Scotts Bluff is just one of several large geological formations along the way that excited the imaginations of road-weary emigrants and served as navigational tools, the way that sailors find their way using the stars. The first rock formations the travelers encountered were Courthouse Rock and Jail Rock that stood out for miles on the monotonous plain, prompting many emigrants to sketch them or, at the very least, write about them in their journals and letters home. Chimney Rock, probably the most famous of the formations, is still an impressive sight despite being slowly whittled away by 150 years of erosion. It marked the end of the Great Plains and the beginning of the slow, but steady climb into the Rocky Mountains. Many emigrants carved their names in the base of Chimney Rock, but we were intimidated by all the signs warning about rattle snakes so we didn't walk up close enough to read the names.

I had read that wagon ruts along the California-Oregon Trail are still visible in a few locations, and I did not want to go home until I saw some. Of course, most of the old trail along the Platte River Valley followed dirt paths on the prairie so that erosion, along with twentieth century development, obliterated most of the traces. Other places have signs indicating that underneath all the present day vegetation and trees, a close observer might be able to discern the remnants of wagon ruts. But in eastern Wyoming, just a few miles beyond Fort Laramie, I was thrilled to see the definitive and amazing Guernsey Ruts where emigrant wagons were forced by the rocky terrain to follow a single, narrow path over the soft sandstone, eventually carving ruts so deep that they are clearly visible more than 150 years later.

Quite a few of the early emigrants did keep journals to record their experiences, and fortunately, some of them have found their way into print because their descendants had the foresight to recognize their significance and often turned them over to universities or historical societies. At Fort Kearny, I bought some books about the California Trail that include diary entries describing the rigors of overland travel in the 1850's. The pioneers were up before dawn to prepare breakfast, pack up their supplies, harness the mules or oxen, and round up the cattle before starting out for the day. Around noon, they stopped to prepare their mid-day meal cooked over a fire of buffalo chips that had to be collected along the way since dry wood was scarce on the virtually treeless prairie. It was also important to allot enough time for the animals to graze and drink their fill of water. In almost every diary entry that I read, drinkable water and grass for the animals were the most important considerations. Without those two necessities, the whole endeavor would fail so experienced trail guides or books written by earlier emigrants were essential for planning the route.

The Platte River and plentiful grass near the rock formations made them popular places for the travelers to make camp for a night or two so the livestock could rest and graze while the men made repairs to the wagons and women took care of their domestic chores. One diarist wrote about baking bread, cookies and biscuits, washing her family's clothes in the river and even doing the ironing!

Babies and the frail elderly were the only people who rode in the wagons. Everyone else had to walk, usually an average of 15 to 20 miles a day, over rocky terrain and through dozens of streams and rivers. Nowhere in my research was I able to find out how many pairs of boots the typical emigrant wore out on the 2,000 mile journey, but I did learn that many people bought moccasins from the Indians along the way to replace their ragged footwear.

The old movie westerns that my generation grew up watching painted a very unfair image of the Native Americans. We were led to believe that attacks by hostile Indians, who liked nothing better than slaughtering white people for their scalps, was the greatest danger the emigrants faced. Actually, wagon accidents, gun mishaps caused by people inexperienced with firearms and cholera were the biggest causes of death along the trail, and many diary entries mentioned the fresh graves the emigrants passed each day. Of the estimated 200,000 emigrants to make the journey in the mid 1800's, 10% died along the way.

Aunt Mollie also recounted a run-in Sarah had with some of Brigham Young's men as they crossed through Mormon Territory. Sarah was a petite red-haired girl who caught the eye of Brigham Young's men who wanted to take her with them. I'm sure there was a shortage of attractive women out there at that time so it seems plausible that Aunt Mollie might not have been exaggerating too much when she said that the men offered to buy Sarah from her brother-in-law for what they thought was a fair price. Henry was outraged and refused to sell Sarah which resulted in a gun fight to defend her. A man from the wagon train was killed in the melee and Henry insisted that Sarah hide her red hair under a big bonnet and stay out of sight as much as possible until they were out of Mormon Territory. She said he was so angry with her for causing trouble that he openly wished he had left her back in Iowa.

The journey from Iowa to California took four months, and when they reached San Francisco, Annie seemed to be much better. However, so many people were flooding into San Francisco thinking the streets were paved with gold, only to be disappointed, that Henry became disenchanted after a few years and decided they should cross back over the Sierra Nevada Mountains to the Nevada territory. On the side of a steep mountain, just twenty miles from the California border, prospectors had discovered what would be known as the Comstock Lode, the greatest silver strike in history. Word traveled fast, luring a big wave of settlers in the late 1850's.

They settled first in White Pine, but soon moved to Virginia City where Henry opened a saddle and harness business like he'd had back in Iowa. Sometime after they were happily settled in Virginia City, Annie gave birth to their first child and then suddenly died. Not too long afterwards, the baby also died and Henry told Sarah that it wouldn't be proper for her to continue living in his house now that his wife was gone so she would have to either find a husband or return to her parents in Iowa.

In one letter from Aunt Mollie, she said that Marco, "the richest, most eligible bachelor in Virginia City," proposed at Annie's wake, but that seems rather ill-mannered, or else crassly opportunistic. It also was another example of Aunt Mollie's embroidery of the truth since there were many very wealthy men on the Comstock Lode. At any rate, they were married on June 16, 1865, by Father

Patrick Manogue in Saint Mary's in the Mountains Roman Catholic Church. Among the wedding guests was John W. Mackay, a Comstock multi-millionaire who gave Marco and Sarah two bronze statues of medieval knights. Aunt Mollie had them in her Butte apartment after her grandparents died and then my mother brought them to our house in Metuchen.

6

When Marco had first arrived in San Francisco in 1853, his plan wasn't to mine gold himself. He was an early entrepreneur who had the financial resources to buy and sell real estate in a city where new businesses were popping up overnight, like mushrooms after a heavy rain. He started a chain of stores catering to the needs of all the new settlers in the rapidly growing city. He had a fruit store at 115 Market Street and a coffee saloon on Market, as well as another fruit store at Kearney and Dupont streets. It's amazing what details you can learn on Google. They even have an inventory list from one of Marco's stores showing he sold much more than fruit.

Silver was discovered in the Nevada territory so he moved to White Pine, Nevada and then Virginia City where he opened the San Francisco Fruit Store and organized the Medin Gold and Silver Mining Company. He also owned several saloons in Virginia City and Hamilton, including the venerable establishments where gentlemen could afford to pay 25 cents for a beer and a game of billiards, down to some lower-end bars catering to poorly-paid laborers.

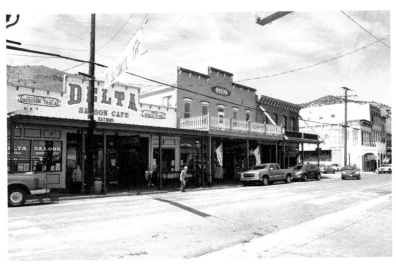

The Delta Saloon is still operating where Marco Medin had one of his saloons in the 1860s and 70's in Virginia City, Nevada. (Photo by the author)

He was a member of the Fat Man's Baseball Club of White Pine, consisting of 21 members whose combined weight added up to 4,856 pounds. Marco weighed in at 240 pounds.

I suspect that Sarah was a little lonely living in a bustling mining town filled primarily with single men and women of easy virtue while her entrepreneurial husband was always busy finding new business opportunities to invest in because she wrote home to her family in Burlington, Iowa and invited her younger sister Maggie to come west for an extended visit. Maggie was about to leave Burlington by overland stage in 1867 when her father Anthony read that Indians had attacked a stagecoach and there were no survivors. Anthony decided the safest route would be by sailing vessel so she went to New

Orleans where she embarked on a voyage around Cape Horn that lasted several months.

During the trip, an Englishman on his way to San Francisco became attracted to the pretty young woman and wrote to her insistently after the trip in care of her sister and brother-in-law in Virginia City. But Sarah had other plans for her little sister and discreetly destroyed the letters. It turns out Marco had a very good friend, Mark Lovely (originally Ljubisich), a fellow Dalmatian from Ragusa. Mark Lovely was also a very wealthy businessman who owned the Silver Age Saloon as well as several mining interests throughout Nevada, and Sarah decided he would be a perfect husband for Maggie, despite his being twice her age.

Years later, Mark Lovely told his grandchildren about taking his bride to Piper's Opera House where everyone turned to admire the petite blonde dressed in a white, crimson-lined cape as she entered by the side of her tall husband. Sarah eventually admitted her duplicitous scheme to keep her sister in Virginia City in a house right next door on South D Street, but by all accounts, Maggie had no complaints and they were happily married for nearly fifty years.

Marco and Sarah had eight children – Antoinette (Tonina, 1866), Marco, Jr., (1868), Sarah (my grandmother who was born in 1870), Joseph (1872), Mamie (1874), Annie (1876), Katherine (1878 who died in childhood) and Tony (1880.) Joseph was born while they were living in Hamilton, Nevada, but he lived for only 18 months. It was soon after Joseph was born that the family traveled back to Budva for a visit in 1873.

Through Ancestry.com I found distant cousins living in Croatia and Slovenia who are also very interested in family history. Olga Medin Srkoc sent me excerpts from a journal written by Marco's cousin Pavao Mikula, a prominent resident of Budva at the time that Marco and Sarah returned in 1873 for a visit. Mikula described Marco and Sarah's four children, two boys and two girls, as "joyful and beautiful," with their mother's fair coloring and a smattering of freckles.

While he was there visiting his family, Marco arranged to have a Catholic chapel built at the old cemetery in Budva. His name in Latin is inscribed over the door.

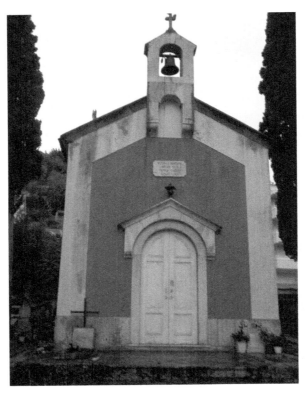

Marco arranged for a Catholic chapel to be built in the old cemetery in Budva. (photo by Olga Srkoc)

Cousin Olga, who now lives in Zagreb, sent me photos of the chapel in Budva where the family still owns the old Medin house within the ancient city walls. Olga's great grandfather Joseph was born 2 years after Marco, but he stayed back in Budva while his brothers expanded the family businesses in America.

Again, through the magic of a Google search, Marco Medin's name appeared in an 1875 travel journal, **_Rambles in Istria, Dalmatia and Montenegro_** by R.H.R, a wealthy man who met Marco when he was passing through Budva in 1873. The author, who I am guessing might have been from the British aristocracy, but wanted to remain somewhat anonymous, wrote, "*At one o'clock a.m., we reached the gates of Budua, where I was met by Baron Heydeg and Signor Marco Medin. Heydeg was an officer quartered with his regiment at Budua, whose acquaintance I had made at Pola, and with whom I had subsequently travelled. Medin was a native of Budua, who had left his country many years before, had made money in California, had married there a buxom Irish girl, a native of Ballinrobe, and had now returned, a rich man, to end his days among his relations in Dalmatia. They had been waiting for me a long time, and had walked some miles on the road to Cattaro to meet me, but were beginning to think I was not going to keep my word.*

We were soon seated together at a comfortable supper, and at half-past two a.m., I was finally allowed to retire to my bed, which Medin had kindly procured for me in a private house – because here, as in Cattaro, there is no hotel of any kind.

Tired and sleepy as I was, I passed but an indifferent night, for, notwithstanding that my room had two large windows overlooking the sea, and that I kept them both open, the heat was perfectly stifling.

I was just thinking of going out the next morning about ten, when in walked the Baron and Signor Medin, and we at once adjourned for breakfast at the same place where we had supped the previous night; I say place, as it was neither an inn nor a café. How shall I describe it? The following is the way we got at it, anyhow. In the main street of Budua, near to the land gate, on the left hand as you come in, you meet with five rugged stone steps, flanked by a shakey single iron railing. These lead up to a strong wooden door, which at some period of its existence may have enjoyed the privilege of paint, but of which no trace remains at the present moment, not even enough to enable one to make a guess at the colour it once enjoyed.

Entering by this door, I found myself in a stuffy, dirty hall, "a terreno," pervaded by a multitude of vile smells, one more awful than the other, but all so dovetailed and commingled that it was perfectly impossible to tell what the composition was. Turning sharp to the left, we mounted a steep stone staircase, at the top of which we were greeted by the same odour that had met us on entering, in which now the smell of assafoetida and garlic clearly predominated. We found ourselves in the kitchen of the establishment, over which reigned supreme a good-humoured, fat German Frau of fifty or more, assisted by two bright-eyed, sharp-looking Dalmatian lads, begrimed with dirt and shining with grease and perspiration. The Frau piloted us through this kitchen, where the heat must have been 110 degrees, if not more, and brought us into the dining-room, a pretty good-sized room with windows round the three sides of it, the furniture consisting solely of one long deal table down the middle, and a score of rush-bottomed chairs around it. At this table were seated a dozen or so of German officers demolishing their "early bit."

I was here received by the Frau's worse half, a portly man of sixty or thereabouts. His coat was off, but he had on instead a huge pair of silver spectacles. He at once showed me to my seat at the table, when I apologized, through the Baron, to the officers for disturbing them at their breakfast.

Notwithstanding the unpromising condition of things, the breakfast was excellent; but mine host in shirt sleeves, with whom I kept up a running conversation in Italian, was even better. ...He was a most amusing character, and combined in himself the functions of doctor, dentist and apothecary, as well as that of keeper of a restaurant in Budua – hence the villainous combination of the odours of a scullery, a kitchen, and a pharmacy.

Having finished our breakfast, Heydeg and I strolled outside the walls to where the market is held under some magnificent old carob trees, and there, as at Cattaro, were numbers of Montenegrins disposing of their produce. Here we had some delicious fresh figs, and then lighting our cigars we went round the old fortifications, which are now only just sufficient for protection at night against any sudden incursion of the wild tribes of the interior. Then we had a good bathe in a most delicious little cove, entirely girt round with rocks, and with a sandy bottom that felt like velvet under our feet. We then again lit another cigar, and started on a tour of exploration through this old town.

Budua, situated at the extreme end of Dalmatia, in what used to be called Northern Albania, is the last Austrian city on the coast of the Adriatic. It is built on a low rocky promontory, and possesses no interest, save in its picturesque appearance, which it derives from its medieval walls and machicolated towers – useless, indeed against a civilized enemy, but still offering some protection from possible irruptions from Albanian freebooters. It is especially picturesque as seen from the sea, with its rugged background of naked mountains. Immediately about it there is some cultivation on the narrow strip of land which lies between the mountains and the sea; and corn, vines, olive trees, and mulberries for the rearing of silk-worms, are diligently grown.

Inside, it is not attractive – its streets are extremely narrow, no more than six feet wide in many instances; they are, however, well paved and would do well enough, were it not for the utter disregard to cleanliness and drainage. Still, there are some wealthy people living there, and many of the houses are very good and substantial. There are several good shops, (perhaps the word stores would best describe them), where a brisk trade seemed to be carried on. The Baron and I poked our way through all the nooks and crannies of the place. We found nothing to invite attention, but a great deal to shock the sight, and even the sense of smell. So we hurried on and went to pay a visit to my buxom Ballinrobe friend, who had not only quite forgotten her ancestral brogue, but had actually exchanged it for a decided American accent, which, to my ears, was not an improvement. She offered us neither English tea nor Irish whiskey punch, but gave us some delicious lemonade and maraschino; and showed by her manner that, if the brogue was gone, the hearty Irish welcome was there still."

7

Aunt Mollie said that just before Marco and Sarah were married, he asked her to return to Europe with him to help him care for his "vast estates." Sarah promised to live there if that was what he wanted but admitted years later to her granddaughter that she had no intention of living anywhere but in America. Apparently, they traveled back to Budva several times, but never stayed for more than long visits. When Mollie admonished her grandmother for not keeping her promise, Sarah just laughed and said, "Promises and pie crust were made to be broken!"

After reading the vivid description of Budva in *"Rambles in Istria, Dalmatia and Montenegro,"* and then seeing it first-hand when Bruce and I hired a driver to take us there from Dubrovnik, I can see why she was reluctant to make her home there permanently. Although the small medieval city is charming and picturesque, it is also decidedly claustrophobic with its narrow streets and high walls. Sarah was now accustomed to the wide open vistas of the American west coupled with a vibrant social mobility that was unheard of in the old cities of Europe. As a compromise, Marco and Sarah returned to his homeland every few years and they sent their three oldest children, ages 7, 5 and 3, to be educated for a time in Dubrovnik (then Ragusa) – Antoinette and Sarah attended a Catholic convent school and Marco, Jr. went to the Jesuit school in the beautiful, old walled city to study Croatian and Italian. Mollie said that Marco's mother was angry with him for abandoning his betrothed and marrying an Irish girl so he had agreed to send his three oldest children back to Europe to be educated to appease her. It must have broken Sarah's heart to leave them behind when she and Marco sailed home to America. Perhaps they had worked out their own compromise because the three youngest children were educated at a school in Virginia City. As the town quickly evolved from a rough mining camp to a civilized little city with churches and an opera house and where families would want to raise their children, the residents built an excellent school that was just a short walk from the Medin's house. When we visited Virginia City in 2013, the school building was still there only now it's an historical center.

Mollie also said that Marco's vast estate included a 100-room hunting lodge with a private suite for when Emperor Franz Joseph came to visit. That stretched my capacity for belief to the extent that I chose not to even mention it until our visit to Zagreb, Croatia in 2016 to meet my cousin Olga Medin Srkoc and her husband Miljenko who had graciously invited us to stay with them in their lovely home. Olga said there definitely was a lodge, but she doubted it had 100 rooms and she was quite certain that the emperor had never come to visit. The Medin family had been prepared to be hospitable should Franz Joseph ever decide to go hunting in Budva, but apparently there were more than enough hunting lodges within the huge Austro-Hungarian Empire to satisfy his needs.

Olga is a retired dentist and Miljenko is a civil engineer with his own structural design firm. Their beautiful daughter Lana is a lawyer and their younger daughter

Tamara, who we didn't have an opportunity to meet, is an orthodontist. Over delicious meals that Olga prepared for us, we shared what we know about our family history and also ventured into some lively discussions of contemporary world politics. The whole family speaks fluent English, and they are much better informed about world events than the average insular American. We enjoyed our visit with them immensely and wished we could have stayed longer, but we were meeting friends in Paris for a river cruise down the Rhone.

~

In 1869, the Nevada Supreme Court was called upon to settle a law suit against Marco that had been festering in the lower courts for most of the decade. Marco and his business partners, mostly men of Dalmatian background, jointly owned several saloons in Virginia City. On July 4, 1863, a partner named Marco Millenovich was shot during an altercation in the *San Francisco Saloon*. To those of us who grew up watching old westerns on television, this kind of thing supposedly happened quite frequently. As his friend and business partner, Marco Medin arranged for the best medical care available at the time in an effort to save the man's life. For ten days, Millenovich struggled to survive and during that time, he asked Marco to send his body back to the city of San Francisco, in the event that his wounds proved to be fatal.

I don't know if Millenovich already had a will in which Marco was designated the executor, or if the legal document was drawn up as he lay on his death bed. But the poor man died from his gunshot wounds and Marco arranged to have Millenovich's body transported back to

San Francisco in a dignified and proper conveyance, as close to a hearse as he could find.

Soon after the will was probated, Millenovich's beneficiaries took exception to the way Marco fulfilled his duties as executor and sued him. One of their complaints was that Marco had spent too much money on Millenovich's funeral and transporting his body in a private vehicle instead of using one of the public carts traveling back and forth between Nevada and California on a weekly basis. It was July in the high desert of Nevada, and I'm guessing that Marco wanted to give his friend a proper burial as quickly as possible. If the beneficiaries had had their way, they probably would have just slung the body over the back of a mule for the journey, figuring Millenovich wouldn't know the difference.

The beneficiaries' greed caused them to nit-pick over almost every aspect of Marco's handling of the estate and, as I read through the legal document, the claimants' clever attorney was making what appeared to be a pretty good case against Marco, except for their whining about the cost of the funeral arrangements. By the time I finished wading through the legal arguments, full of circumlocuitous jargon, I was pleased to find that the judges concluded that… "we find nothing in the record to impeach either the good faith or the judgement of the executor…." Aside from being pleased for Marco's sake, I was very impressed with how quickly this brand new, sparsely populated state had put together all the working parts of a civil society.

~

During the 1870's Samuel Clemens was working as a reporter on *The Territorial Enterprise* whose offices were located directly across the street from one of Marco's saloons and a few doors down from his store that sold fine cigars and imported whiskey, among other things. Marco had a quick wit and was known as a jovial story teller so it's not too far out of the realm of possibility to think that he and Sam Clemens might have smoked some cigars while exchanging some tall tales over a drink on occasion. It was during his time in Virginia City that Clemens adopted the pen name of Mark Twain and his book, ***Roughing It,*** published in 1872, was a semi-autobiographical collection of travel stories about his time in the American west.

Virginia City, like most cities and towns across the United States, was filled with wooden structures, built close together and then put at great risk by the use of candles, oil lamps, wood stoves, careless people and inadequate fire-fighting equipment. From 1860 to 1880, the town and nearby Gold Hill suffered numerous fires which destroyed entire residential and business areas.

On October 26, 1875, fire broke out in a lodging house on A Street, resulting in the worst fire in the town's short history as heavy winds swept the flames down the steep hill, from one end of town to the other. In 14 hours, 2,000 buildings were leveled, 10,000 people were left homeless and an estimated $7 million in property was destroyed, a staggering sum in those days. Marco lost ten buildings in the conflagration valued at $150,000, an impressive fortune at that time. Many residents and business owners who lost everything they owned had no insurance, but Marco had $50,000 in coverage and was able to start rebuilding as soon as the charred rubble was hauled away. Their house, fortunately, was located just far enough south of the center of town that they were among the few homeowners to be spared.

Four years later, former president Ulysses S. Grant arrived in town with his wife and son. Following his term in office, Grant and his family had embarked on a two-year trip around the world to see the sites, and everywhere they went, the famous general who had won the Civil War was cheered and feted with banquets and parades. The people of Virginia City were honored that Grant had included their little city on his itinerary. And for his part, Grant wanted to thank the town's residents, and particularly the mine owners and workers, for the silver and gold from the Comstock Lode that helped pay for the Union Army's victory. It was this great wealth dug from the side of Mt. Davidson that had led to Nevada quickly becoming a state in 1864, after only three years as a territory, because President Lincoln and many members of Congress wanted to keep the Comstock silver mines from falling out of Union control and possibly aiding the Confederacy.

An 1879 photo from Grant's visit shows a disheveled group, including President Grant and his wife, along with Nevada Governor Kinkead and silver barons John Mackay and James Fair, posing with lanterns as they emerged from one of the mine shafts. A dinner to honor President Grant had more guests in attendance than any of the local dignitaries and millionaire mine owners could accommodate so several families were asked to loan their fine china and crystal for the occasion. Patriotic Sarah was very happy to oblige.

She told her children that when war broke out between the North and South, she was so angry she wished she could have passed as a man and gone off to fight to save the Union. Two of her brothers were less enchanted by the mythical glory of war and chose to pay other men to take their places in the compulsory draft, as was allowed in the 1863 Conscription Act. From the safe distance of the peaceful Nevada Territory, Sarah was appalled.

I came across a newspaper article from the late 1870's about Marco and Sarah's daughter Antoinette, affectionately called Tonina by her family. The Medins were next door neighbors with the Finlen family who had a newborn baby that Tonina just adored. One day, Mr. and Mrs. Finlen were horrified to discover that their infant, who had been placed in his cradle earlier for a nap, was no longer there. The sheriff was called and the whole neighborhood was enlisted to hunt down the kidnapper and return the precious baby to his parents. It turned out that Tonina, who was maybe 8 or 9 at the time, had sneaked the baby out of the house when all the adults were otherwise engaged and tucked him away in her own bed where she planned to keep him until her parents discovered what she had done. Fortunately, the Finlens were very good friends and, once they knew their baby was safe, were magnanimous enough to find the whole episode very amusing. It makes me wonder, though, what was so intriguing about the Finlen's baby when her own mother produced a new baby for her to play with every two years.

Virginia City society was divided into several different strata. The largest segment of the population was made up of single men working in the mines, and as was often the case in mining towns, the largest occupation for unmarried women on the Comstock was prostitution. There were few opportunities for employment other than doing laundry or domestic work for less than $25 a month so many desperate women turned to the sex trade to support themselves. In 1861, the Nevada Territory had taken the official English Common Law view that brothels were a public nuisance, but not illegal, so a thriving red light district grew up on D Street, just one block east of the central business district.

Not all the prostitutes were viewed with scorn by the townspeople. Julia Bulette, a very popular prostitute, ran a tastefully-furnished high-end establishment where fine wines and liquors were served and clients were required to behave like gentlemen. One bitterly cold January morning, she was found brutally murdered in her little house on the corner of D and Union Streets. Residents of Virginia City were stunned and her friends at Fire Company Number 1purchased a beautiful silver-handled casket and held her funeral in their engine house. After the funeral, a brass band led about 60 firemen and 16 carriages of mourners through a snow storm to her burial place, marked with a simple wooden plank with the name "Julia." Because she was a prostitute, the local churches wouldn't allow her to be buried in sanctified ground so her final resting place sits all alone with her little cross and a fence around the grave to mark the spot. Afterwards, the men marched back into town singing "The Girl I Left Behind," the town was draped in black, and for the first time since President Lincoln's death, all the saloons were closed for the day out of respect.

Rose Benjamin, on the other hand, was known as the most notorious prostitute of Virginia City and had a reputation for being a harsh madam who exploited the often desperate women who worked in her brothel. On one occasion, she was accused of luring a fourteen-year-old girl into her house and giving her opium. As the number of families with children in town grew, it became a little harder to turn a blind eye to the more sordid aspects of the sex trade and the red light district was gradually pushed further away from the more respectable businesses. Rose's brothel on D Street happened to be on a piece of property that Marco owned. By the early 1880's Marco bought them out for $900 and as Rose and her husband George Perkins left town to set up a new brothel in the latest boom town of Butte, Montana, they set fire to their house. No amount of digging into old news articles has revealed if they torched the house to spite Marco or if they were doing him a favor, assuming the property was insured.

While they were still living in Virginia City, Nevada, Sarah's very elderly father Anthony Thornton came to live with them. An old obituary from November 1883 said that he was 107 when he finally died, only the local newspaper reported that "Anthony Torrington, father of Mrs. Marco Medin" had died. Without that tip off, I never would have known my great great grandfather, born the year the American colonies declared independence from Great Britain, had journeyed from Iowa to Nevada and died at such an advanced age. The Irish don't pronounce "h" when it follows "t" and the Irish brogue accounts for the elongation of the "orn" sound. We didn't discover this new bit of family history until after our trip to Virginia City or else we would have spent time in the old cemeteries looking for his grave stone.

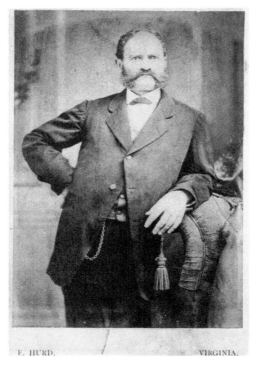

F. HURD.   VIRGINIA.

*Marco Medin, born in 1824 in Budva, Montenegro, came to America
in 1853 and became a pioneer of three states: California, Nevada and
Montana. (F. Hurd Studio, Virginia City, Nevada)*

8

B y the late 1870's, gold, silver and copper were discovered in Butte, Montana so in 1884, Marco and Sarah moved their family north to the "richest hill on earth" where they expanded their businesses. This latest discovery of riches to be had in Butte came at a very fortuitous time because the mines in Virginia City had played out, people were moving out in droves and suddenly Marco's real estate and mining stock were worthless. In a newspaper article of the time, Marco is quoted saying that he left behind $3 million in real estate, including a mansion with French plate glass windows, staircases with carved walnut newel posts, fine large mirrors and massive furniture. "It wouldn't pay to haul them out," he said. Marco had only $10,000 in the bank when they arrived in Butte and opened the Medin Grocery and Fruit Store at 53 West Broadway, across the street from the Butte Opera House. At the age of 62, Marco had made and lost several fortunes so instead of building another elegant home like the one they had in Virginia City, they chose to live in an apartment above their store.

While still in Virginia City, we visited the Storey County Courthouse and studied the old tax assessment maps of the 1860's and 70's to see where Marco and Sarah's house once stood. The address was 188 South D Street, between the Savage Mansion and the Fourth Ward

School. Whether the house was destroyed in a later fire or succumbed to wood rot and vandalism, there is nothing but a weed-filled lot there today.

I don't know how many years Antoinette, Marco, Jr. and Sarah spent going to school in Ragusa (now Dubrovnik), but records show that Antoinette was married to Marco Zarick in Gold Hill, the town next to Virginia City. She and her new husband promptly moved to Sacramento and had a very large family where many of their descendants still live. Sarah and the younger children moved with their parents to Butte, which was becoming a cosmopolitan center with several churches, stores offering a wide variety of consumer goods, a library and the opera house where touring companies would perform as they traveled through the West. Before long, Butte had more Irish people living there than the city of Dublin.

By the time my grandmother Sarah, known as Sadie by her family, completed her education, my grandfather had worked his way up from tool boy in the Alice mine to shift boss at the Green Mountain mine. I would love to know how they met and what their courtship was like since they must have moved in vastly different spheres, with Grandma being a pampered, educated daughter of a fairly wealthy merchant and Grandpa a copper miner with probably no more than an eighth-grade education. That's not to say that he wasn't smart despite his lack of formal schooling and I have no doubt they were very much in love.

Sadie was 21 and John was 26 when they were married on April 15, 1891, around the same time he was made foreman of the mine. Their first child, named Anastasia after his mother back in Ireland, was born in July 1892. Then, two years later, Mary, or Mollie as everyone called her, was born. A promotion to superintendent of the Moonlight mine came just in time as the O'Meara family grew. Two years after Sarah Honore was born in 1896, Senator Millard of Nebraska sent Grandpa to Virginia City, Montana, as general manager of the Kennett mine.

Their first son, John Marco, was born in 1898, but the following year he died from one of the childhood diseases like diphtheria or whooping cough that carried off so many infants before medical science developed a way to immunize babies.

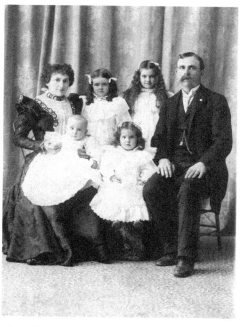

By 1898, Sarah and John O'Meara had 4 children: Anastasia, Mollie, Sarah and John Marco. (Elite Studio, Butte, Montana)

According to Aunt Mollie, in the course of his mining career, Grandpa broke every bone in his body at least once. Although an obvious exaggeration, there were occasional underground explosions and collapsing mine shafts so it seems logical that such a dangerous profession would have led to at least a few serious injuries. Grandma worried constantly and begged him to find another line of work. Perhaps because of her worry, coupled with their grief over their infant son's death, 1899 was the year Grandpa gave up delving into the earth for precious ores and became a brewer, serving as outside manager of the Centennial Brewing Company. After five years, he sold his interests in the Centennial to become secretary and treasurer of the Olympia Brewing Company. Later, he became president of the Olympia and when it was merged with the Centennial, grandpa was selected as manager.

In 1900, Grandma gave birth to their second son, John Medin. Poor little baby John suffered some sort of head trauma that left him so incapacitated that he was sent to live in an institution in Wisconsin where he could be cared for. Aunt Mollie said the nurse dropped him on his head soon after he was born, but knowing the stigma that people felt for any kind of neurological birth defect in those days, it's entirely possible that his affliction wasn't really the result of a careless accident. No one talked about John Medin and my mother never knew she had a brain damaged brother until he died in 1918.

During this time, Grandpa was elected president of the Ancient Order of Hibernians in Montana, a fraternal organization that fostered Irish culture, provided financial assistance to injured or sick members and raised money to send back to the homeland for the Irish Freedom Fund. In *The Butte Irish: Class and Ethnicity in an American Mining Town, 1875 – 1925*, Grandpa was mentioned eleven times for his role as a successful businessman and community leader.

In 1905, Grandpa was on the executive board of the Thomas Francis Meagher Memorial Association, a group of Irish patriots who raised $10,000 for a bronze statue to honor the exiled Irish revolutionary and first governor of the Montana Territory. A native of Grandpa's home county of Waterford, Meagher had been accused of high treason by the British government and sentenced to be strung and quartered. Possibly fearing a violent backlash by the Irish citizenry, Meagher was banished to Tasmania, instead. He somehow managed to escape in 1852 and arrived in New York by 1855 where he practiced law and was active in the Irish independence movement. With the outbreak of the Civil War, he organized a band of Zouaves and fought at the first battle of Bull Run. Later, he organized what became known as the Irish Brigade and served with distinction at the Battle of Fredericksburg. In 1866, at the recommendation of General Grant, Meagher was appointed acting governor of Montana, but he served for only about a year before falling off a boat near Fort Benton and drowning in the Missouri River. Some say he had been drinking. It was a sad end to a noble career, but the Irish were very proud of him and Grandpa was doubly proud when his 13-year-old daughter Anastasia was selected to unveil Meagher's statue at the state capital of Helena. An identical statue stands outside the Tower Hotel in the city of Waterford.

Like most of the towns in the West, Butte was a city populated almost exclusively by recent immigrants. At one point, as I noted earlier, Butte had more Irish living there than Dublin. Many of the immigrants planned to work hard for several years, make as much money as possible and then return home to live out their lives in relative prosperity. Grandpa's younger brother Michael and one of his older half-brothers did that. Quite possibly, that might have even been my grandfather's original intent, but once he married my grandmother, who was born in America, bought a house and started a family, he had laid down roots that were hard to pull up. There were two Irish camps in Butte – those whose first loyalty was to the Irish motherland and those who still deeply loved Ireland, but were committed to being American first. There were several references in ***The Butte Irish*** to things Grandpa said and that his fellow Hibernians said about him, that show he was conflicted in his loyalties. Perhaps if his aging parents weren't still back in Ireland struggling to earn a living on their tiny farm while waiting for the financial assistance their children periodically sent back from Butte, and if the country weren't still suffering under the oppressive rule of Great Britain, Grandpa could have settled comfortably into his new status as an American without any lingering pangs of guilt.

~

On June 24, 1901, Marco Medin died suddenly at the age of 77. His obituary, which lavishly praised him as a pioneer of three states, attributed his death to old age. Five days later, his twenty-five-year-old daughter Annie committed suicide by swallowing carbolic acid. The *San Francisco Chronicle* wrote, "Mrs. Annie O'Brien, a prominent society woman, the wife of William O'Brien, an architect, died this evening under circumstances that point strongly to suicide while mentally deranged... Today the father's will was filed for probate, and it was found he had left all his large estate to the widow. This is supposed to have preyed upon Mrs. O'Brien's mind. The coroner's jury returned a verdict of accidental death."

I doubt that my mother even knew that her aunt, who had died nine years before she was born, had committed suicide. And why would the fact that her father left his estate to her mother, a normal occurrence in most families, be a reason to take her own life?

Right around this time, my grandparents left Butte for three months to visit his mother Anastasia and his younger brother Michael back in Bunmahon. His father John J. O'Meara, Sr. had died in 1898 and I'm sure he must have regretted not returning home sooner. They brought their three daughters who were nine, seven and five at the time and Mollie's most vivid impression of her grandmother was that she had a naturel "marcel" wave in her hair. During this visit, they bought several large pieces of Waterford crystal that my mother eventually inherited and kept on display in the dining room. When we were children, Mark and I had been warned so many times not to play near them and risk breaking these family treasures that I figured if I ever did accidentally break one of them, it would be best to just leave home and not come back.

After twenty-one years away, my grandfather must have been so proud to return home as a successful businessman with a wife and three children, while at the same time, my grandmother must have been wretched with guilt for leaving her mother so soon after the deaths of her father and sister. Soon after they returned from Ireland, the Butte society pages reported that Sarah Medin and her daughter Mamie Holland were spending the winter in California, and my grandparents were moving into Sarah's home in her absence.

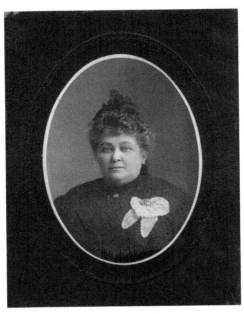

Sarah Thornton Medin, came to America at the age of 6 in 1845, traveled to California by wagon train at the age of 16, during the great westward migration, then moved to Nevada where she met and married Marco Medin and ended her days in Butte, Montana.

A few months later, Marco and Sarah's son, Marco, Jr. eloped with a young woman he met over the telephone. The headline in the *Salt Lake Herald* snickered "Marco is Rich; Alice is Fair – And Stern Papa McManus is Up in the Air." Marco was recently divorced from his first wife Celia and had been awarded custody of their little boy Marco Medin III. The newspaper described the romance like this, "Miss McManus is very pretty. She has a jolly nice voice, too. It was the voice which caught Marco first. Miss McManus was a "helloo" girl in the central [phone company] office at Butte. Marco runs a wine house and general grocery store on West Broadway, and has occasion to use the telephone frequently. It was while talking to customers he got acquainted with that voice, and he was captured by it. He pursued the matter further and became acquainted with the young woman. He thought her just as sweet as her voice, and paid lavish attention to her.

"All this was agreeable to the young woman, but not to old George. He did not like Marco, although the latter is one of the handsomest men in all Butte, and so, when the young merchant applied for the hand of the young woman, George told him plainly he would have none of it."

The article went on to describe how Marco arrived to take Alice out for an innocent walk, which her father thought was harmless enough, not knowing that Marco had a marriage license in his pocket and they had a local judge perform the ceremony that afternoon. Later that night, while George McManus was sleeping, unaware that his daughter was married, Marco and his friends sneaked into the McManus house to get Alice's trunk and the two newlyweds boarded a train for a wedding trip to Salt Lake City. The article concluded that Papa McManus would eventually relent and give the couple his blessing. "If he does not, it will make no difference, for Marco is rich, and is the manager of a vast estate left by his father who died last summer, leaving behind him lots of real estate and money in the bank."

Alice must have been quite an exceptional beauty because seven years later, after a quick divorce from Marco, she married the younger son of the obscenely-rich copper baron and former senator William A. Clark. William, Jr. fell in love with Alice at first sight and married her only a few days after they met.

Marco tried a stint at mining gold in Alaska, but failed at that and quickly returned home. Unfortunately, he made the newspapers again in 1912 when he was arrested for selling liquor to two underage girls, one of whom claimed to be nineteen but was actually only fourteen.

A few years later, Marco married a third time to Mabel Reins, daughter of a Butte physician, but that marriage also ended in divorce and Mabel died in a car accident in Los Angeles in 1942.

I imagine my proper grandmother Sadie was quite mystified by her older brother Marco's lifestyle, but meanwhile, her own life with my grandfather continued in a proper Catholic trajectory. In 1903, their son Harney was born and named in honor of his paternal grandmother Anastasia's maiden name. Two years later, Francis Xavier was born, only to die shortly after his first birthday.

By 1909, Grandma was pregnant again and Anastasia and Mollie, who were in their mid-teens, were mortified. Their stern disapproval of such "old" people still being sexually active was so palpable that Grandma was in tears and Grandpa was furious. After much discussion, my grandparents decided to ship their two older daughters off to the Convent of the Visitation, a cloistered convent boarding school in Georgetown, Washington, until after the birth of my mother Eileen Virginia on January 12, 1910. Sarah, who was 14 at the time and would become my mother's favorite sister because of her sweet, loving nature, was looking forward to having a baby to play with. Anastasia, 18, and Mollie, 16, became resigned to the inevitable and actually grew to love their little sister who they stuck with the nickname "Baby" until she was well into her fifties.

9

When I was a child, I enjoyed looking through my mother's old Kodak book, filled with faded black & white photos of a family I had heard stories about but never met. In those days, before amateur flash photography, most of the family photos were taken out on the front porch of their Dutch colonial house at 307 West Granite Street. Looking back now, I remember thinking everyone looked sad in those old photos. It wasn't until recently that I realized people rarely ever smiled when their picture was taken, either because it wasn't the fashion back then or, possibly, they were self-conscious about their teeth. But maybe even more than that, black & white photography made it look as though everyone was dressed in mourning when in reality, my fashionable grandmother and aunts were probably dressed in a multitude of lovely colors. But perhaps my perception was shaded most by the stories my mother had told me about the flu pandemic and the financial hardship the family faced after her parents' death.

But now that my mother's memory had receded far back into her childhood, she seemed to have settled on the years before 1918 when the house was filled with the sounds of dinner parties and beaux calling on her older sisters. She, too, enjoyed looking at these old photos again of her beloved Mama and Papa and her sisters and brother.

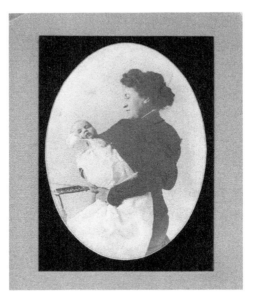

Sarah Medin O'Meara holding her eighth and final child, Eileen Virginia O'Meara. (Photo by the Gibson Studio, Butte, Montana)

The album opens with photos of my mother as an infant in her mother's arms and others showing the family dressed in what was probably their Sunday finery. My grandmother Sarah and her teenage daughters Anastasia, Mollie and Sarah are all very elegantly turned out in the long dresses and large plumed hats that were stylish in 1910, before the revolutionary change that ushered in short skirts and bobbed hair.

Another photo shows the family in a very large car that seems to have enough seats for 3 rows of passengers. It belonged either to my grandfather or to his brother-in-law Marco who had made his fortune in road paving as automobiles were quickly replacing horse-drawn carriages. Grandma is wearing an enormous hat festooned with feathers and tied to her head so it wouldn't blow off while riding in the open vehicle. In the next photo, Uncle Harney, age 8, was sitting in the driver's seat sulking with what I imagine was probably acute disappointment at being told he couldn't drive.

When I looked through her Kodak book with a fresh eye, I noticed for the first time a tent pitched on the porch roof and remembered my mother telling me her brother Harney used to pretend he was camping outside his bedroom window. There was a decorative railing around the porch roof creating a balcony effect and a row of flower boxes in front of the railing as well as along the porch below it. Flowers and vinca vine cascaded down the front of the house making what must have been a colorful display.

The wide porch had a swing at one end and some of the photos show four-year-old Eileen, who would eventually become my mother, sitting on it with the family spaniel or with her father, dressed in a three-piece suit with a gold watch chain stretched over his prosperous-looking belly, all the while looking vaguely distracted for some reason. Her brother Harney is dressed in knickers and smiling impishly at the camera as he dangles some books bound together with a belt, making this, possibly, a first-day-of-school photo. Another photo shows a group of people, most of them women, sitting in chairs on the front porch. One of them must be Great-grandma Sarah Medin because she is so much older and stouter than everyone else and has a stern expression on her face. My mother remembered her as being crabby and not very patient by the time she knew her, although Aunt Mollie, sixteen years older than my mother, had an entirely different recollection of life with Grandma Medin who had experienced many exciting adventures when she was young and had found an avid listener in her granddaughter Mollie.

There are pictures of birthday parties with neighborhood children in front of an elaborate play house out on "the Five Mile" where many Butte families had vacation homes and others showing a six-year-old Eileen wearing a poke bonnet to protect her fair skin from the sun while playing with her friends in the backyard sand pile.

To escape the long, harsh Montana winters, the O'Meara family spent the month of February in San Diego, staying at the famous Hotel del Coronado. They packed up the steamer trunks, the ones that had traveled across country several times to boarding school and to Ireland and back, with enough dresses and hats to last a month. In every picture, the family is elegantly turned out in the latest fashion, including the knee-length dresses modest young women wore at the beach if they planned to take a dip in the water. My grandmother, however, was always dressed in a dignified outfit, suitable for a woman in her mid-forties, although she would at least remove her wide-brimmed hat so her face could be seen in the group photos on the beach. She always looked to me like a stern dowager casting a pall over the family fun, but my mother had such wonderful memories of a loving, attentive mother presiding over happy family gatherings that I'm sure now her photographs didn't reflect her true personality.

During one of their trips to San Diego when my mother was five, the whole family went on an outing to the border with Mexico. The photo shows my grandparents, mother, Anastasia, Sarah, Harney and Mollie lined up in front of a 1915 touring car holding two banners that said "On the Boundary Line" and "US & Mex." They were so well dressed, they could have been heading off to church or a garden party.

One of my favorite pictures shows my eight-year-old mother, her long hair blowing in the breeze, standing on the Coronado Hotel beach with a boy she described as her first "beau." His name was Henry Wheeler and he stood there with his arm around her shoulder with an air of masculine confidence.

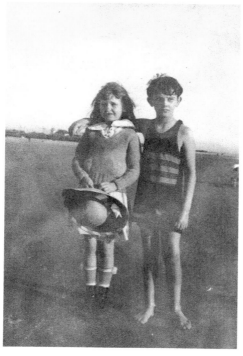

Eileen at 8 years old, on the Hotel del Coronado beach with her first "beau" Henry Wheeler. (Photo by Mollie O'Meara, 1918)

Another photo shows my mother, a big bow in her hair and tassels decorating her knee socks, and Henry dressed in knickers with a matching tweed jacket, taking a break from roller skating around the hotel grounds to pose for pictures. Henry was the one who introduced my mother to L. Frank Baum's Wizard of Oz series of books which were the rage among children back then. He was the son of a wealthy divorcee from New York who liked to spend her winters in San Diego. Henry had met Baum and had given the author an enthusiastic critique of Dorothy's adventures in Oz. His enthusiasm was so contagious that my mother never got over it and continued into adulthood to reread *The Wonderful Wizard of Oz* and all 13 of the sequels whenever she felt the need to escape the real-life worries that were dragging her down.

Knowing what was to happen to this happy family in just eight short months, my eyes sometimes fill with tears, even now, when I look at these faded pictures of them playing on the beach, my mother buried up to her neck in the sand and grinning at the camera or dancing on the hotel lawn in a ballet costume her mother had made for her to wear to the Valentine's Day costume party.

Upon closer inspection of the photos, I realized I had missed one showing my grandmother, rather formally dressed for sitting in the sand, but smiling joyfully at her children.

My mother's favorite photographs, however, were the formal portraits of her parents that I found up in the attic when I was cleaning out her house. They were taken by Count Matzene, a well-known photographer in the early years of the Twentieth Century, who specialized in artistic portraiture, particularly of women.

Because Matzene felt that pose was most significant as an expression of personality, he favored images in which the whole body or substantial portions were visible and he emphasized the quality of the sitters' clothing. I had the two portraits framed and hung them in her assisted living apartment where she could gaze at them throughout the day and be reminded of happier times. The portraits were taken in 1917, the year before the big flu pandemic when everything changed.

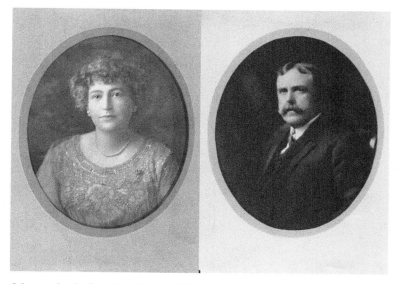

My mother's favorite photos of her parents were the formal portraits taken in 1917, the year before the great flu pandemic killed 50 million people worldwide and brought tragedy to her family. (Matzene, Butte, Montana)

10

When my mother was fifteen, she was sent to Washington to attend the Convent of the Visitation, the same elite private school in Georgetown that her three older sisters had attended, but this time she was a scholarship student.

Even though the convent was cloistered and the students weren't allowed to leave the campus without an appropriate chaperone, my mother was very happy there. First of all, she was away from her quarreling older sisters who had breezed through their inheritance and couldn't pay the bills. It wasn't entirely their fault, however, since they had been raised to do fancy needlework, arrange flowers, visit the dressmaker and attend lovely parties. They had been groomed to marry well and preside over a comfortable home, not earn a living. My grandfather seemed to feel it would reflect badly upon his role as a loving father if he expected his daughters to support themselves. Mollie, at least, had rebelled and had managed to persuade her father to allow her to attend Columbia University where she was preparing for a teaching career when she was suddenly summoned home by her father just before he died.

Anastasia had been doing something vaguely described as "war work" in Washington, D.C. It was 1918 and the world was rapidly changing, so much so, that this gently-reared graduate of a cloistered convent school was now living on her own in the big city and enjoying the unchaperoned company of a variety of young gentlemen. Anastasia had to interrupt her exciting social life to rush back home when she received the telegram about the sudden death of her mother and sister Sarah and the precarious condition of her father. Anastasia, Mollie and Harney arrived home just in time to say goodbye to their father who had seemed to be recovering before suffering a fatal relapse of the deadly virus. Mollie always said it was a broken heart that killed him, not the flu. The story of three members of the same family all dying within days of each other was so tragic, it made the front pages of all the newspapers in Montana.

Death Enters the O'Meara Household – *City's Sympathy Goes out to Stricken Family* - *Saturday, October 26, 1918*

"There is scarcely another event in the whole history of our city so sad as the terrible tragedy which during the week befell the respected and now widely mourned family of the late Mr. and Mrs. John J. O'Meara, three members of one family, all of them in the full glow of health only a few weeks ago – dead within a few brief days of each other – first the mother – gentle, tender, noble matron, then the daughter – stainless in all the simple innocence of maidenhood and finally the father – brave, upright, courageous man. Yea a few weeks ago this family, socially among the very foremost of our city, was happy in the enjoyment of health and the esteem of their fellow citizens; and then like a bolt from a clear sky the depopulating epidemic that, with pestilential fury is sweeping over the face of this land, entered their happy household and from Saturday afternoon till Tuesday morning the Grim Reaper Death seemed ready to devour all of that once blessed and contented family....only

four orphan children left to mourn the loss of an ideal mother, a devoted father and a sweetly, tender sister."

John J. O'Meara Follows Wife and Child to Grave – Prominent Butte Business Man Unable to Withstand Ravages of Influenza. End Comes at Hour Set for Double Funeral

John J. O'Meara, manager of the Centennial Brewing Company and one of Butte's best known citizens, died this morning at 11 o'clock, just at the time when the double funeral of his wife and daughter, Miss Sadie O'Meara, was to have started from the family residence, 307 West Granite Street, to the old Catholic cemetery....

Miss Anastasia O'Meara and Miss Mollie O'Meara, who had been attending war activity schools in New York and Washington, and a son Harney, who had been a member of the students' training camp at Georgetown University, arrived in the city last evening in response to telegrams as to the serious illness of mother and sister, only to find both dead and the father critically ill. The three crowded about the bedside of their father and he whispered words of consolation to them. The medical men in attendance pronounced the case of Mr. O'Meara hopeless and the three children never left his bedside during the entire night and not until death came this morning...."

Triple Tragedy *(The Montana American)*

"The triple tragedy of the O'Meara family came with exceptional sorrow to those who were privileged to know the O'Mearas in their almost idealistic home life. Many men knew John O'Meara; only a few knew the father, mother and daughter, and a relatively few knew the unusual and abiding

happiness of a family circle that was shattered in the space of a few days. John O'Meara was a man's man, but with that bold, blunt front of his went a tenderness for those he loved, far removed from the workaday world. He was the gentlest of men with a gracious gentleness that reflected itself in all the members of his family.

"O'Meara was unchanging in his views, uncompromising in his attitudes; bitter in his dislikes, and firm in his friendships. His Americanism might set an example his enemies might have emulated, and with it he stood solidly for justice to Ireland. He stood for it and he talked for it, and he was proud of his attitude. For a half century in this country he never wavered in his righteous defense of the land of his birth, though he stood first, last and all the time for the land of his adoption. The two principles were never in conflict and are only in conflict in the minds of those who neither know nor care about the submerging and suppression of small races and nations. Write it above O'Meara's grave that he loved Ireland. He would have it so.

"There are many tears for Belgium and Servia during the past four years, surely it can not be a crime to have a heart throb for Ireland's ten centuries of wrong. O'Meara was not only intense – he was right.

"In community and civic life he was big and broad; his enterprises existed under the laws of the land and he was a large and free contributor to every philanthropic measure for public good, even in the hours when his fortunes were being confiscated by prohibitionists.

"Death came with triple and unexpected severity, but O'Meara's memory will live long in the hearts of those who knew him as a good man, a good American and one who never wavered in devotion to Ireland."

My poor grandfather never lived to meet Eamon de Valera, President of the Provisional Irish Republic, who visited Butte in 1919 to thank the citizens for their financial support or to see his beloved motherland finally win its full independence from England in 1949.

The newspaper accounts of the triple tragedy described the hundreds of people lined up outside the O'Meara's house on West Granite Street to watch the coffins being carried down the stairs and loaded into the three horse-drawn hearses that would carry them to the old Catholic cemetery. So many flowers were sent to their home that my mother had a lifelong aversion to a scent that only served to remind her of this horrible day.

My mother's brother Harney, who was sixteen at the time and away at Georgetown University's prep school when he was summoned home, was so traumatized by his parents' and sister's sudden deaths that he suffered what was diagnosed as hysterical blindness.

Every Sunday for the next few months, Anastasia and Mollie would take my mother and Harney to the cemetery to pray and pay their respects when my mother knew already, at the age of 8, that since she could never have her parents and sister back, she wanted at least to be allowed to remember them as they had been instead of as three bodies in the cold ground. After my father died in October 1947, never once did she take Mark and me to visit his gravesite, and she loathed fall flowers.

A few months after the funeral, Anastasia, Mollie, Harney and my nine-year-old mother boarded a train for Washington, D.C. to see an eye specialist. There were excellent ophthalmologists in San Francisco, Chicago and New York, but no doubt Anastasia was also eager to get back to her exciting social life. Butte was still a rough mining town so Anastasia and Mollie had the windows of their house boarded up, and an armed guard posted on the front porch every night to keep out thieves. Soon after they left, while the guard was watching vigilantly or, more probably, dozing on the porch, men broke into the house by sliding down the coal chute and stole all the alcohol in my grandfather's wine cellar. That seemed to be all they really cared about because the family silver and other valuables were left behind.

11

The happy family photos in my mother's Kodak book that were taken in February of 1918 at the Hotel del Coronado in San Diego were followed by a gap of a year. Next, we see photos of Anastasia and Mollie in stylish mourning attire posing with Harney and my mother in front of the Wardman Park Hotel where they stayed in Washington, or in front of the Lee mansion in Arlington National Cemetery and other landmarks around the city. An unidentified but distinguished-looking gentleman is standing with them in some of the photos so I'm assuming he was Anastasia's latest beau.

Harney's eyes improved, although for the rest of his life he was considered legally blind. The family returned to Butte, taking the scenic and more expensive route via steamer on the Great Lakes. The 1920's census shows Anastasia listed as head of household but with nothing under occupation. She kept one servant to help run the house and rented out a few rooms to help make ends meet.

My grandfather, unfortunately, had died without a will and his business partners at the brewery apparently weren't as generous as Anastasia and Mollie thought they should be. Before long, bill collectors started appearing at the door and, as Anastasia and Mollie hid behind the draperies, my 10-year-old mother was sent forth to deal with them. Smarting with shame, she had to lie and say her sisters weren't home and, yes, she would give them the message as soon as they returned. When the bill collectors were gone, her sisters would resume their quarreling over money and beaux and the unfair responsibility that had been foisted upon them, and my mother would retreat upstairs to the library to seek solace in the pages of a book.

Somehow, the sisters were able to keep the house and continue to dress fashionably, and Harney was sent off to college and then law school at Georgetown University. Maybe my mother's grandmother and aunts and uncles helped out for a while, but eventually the house had to be sold and that's when my mother was sent east to the Convent of the Visitation in Georgetown, the historic school founded in 1799 where her sisters had gone before her.

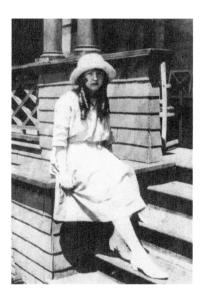

Eileen, age 15, on the front porch of the family home in Butte, shortly before leaving for boarding school in Washington, D.C. (Photo by Harney O'Meara, 1925)

My mother adored the nuns at Georgetown. There were no whippings for minor transgressions or public humiliation meted out for a wrong answer as had happened in her old parochial school back in Butte, causing sensitive children to develop nervous ticks and nightmares. The nuns at Georgetown were from the Salesian tradition and were unlike any nuns she had ever encountered before. They loved their chosen vocation as teachers, nurturing the girls in their care with a deep respect for and joy in learning. My mother's favorite room was the library, lined with floor-to-ceiling bookcases filled with old leather-bound volumes and dark furniture smelling of lemon oil and dust.

The young ladies at the convent were allowed to have gentleman callers on Sunday afternoons. After dinner, the girls waited for their boyfriends in the parlor, the only room in the convent where men were permitted. Self-consciously, the young couples tried to keep their conversations going, knowing there was a nun sitting quietly behind a latticework screen, making sure the discussions didn't veer off into any inappropriate topics. The girls were also permitted to go out with suitable young men, provided they had a chaperone. My mother's beau was a student at Georgetown University, right next door, who had a part time job chauffeuring the Papal Legate on his Sunday afternoon drives out in the countryside. The Papal Legate was a kind, indulgent man who had no objection to his young chauffer bringing his girlfriend along to keep him company in the front seat of the limousine. The nuns were delighted for, other than the Pope himself, who could hope for a better chaperone.

In the 1920's Anastasia was living in the elegant Wardman Park Hotel in Washington, close enough to

Embassy Row that many of her neighbors were wealthy, high level men in the diplomatic corp, just the kind of people with whom she especially loved to spend time. When my mother was in her senior year of high school, Anastasia would sweep into the convent on weekends, and with the nuns unwitting permission, take my mother out for the day to attend luncheons and parties where she could introduce her beautiful little sister to her influential friends.

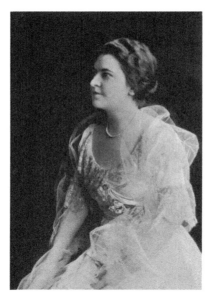

My mother's oldest sister Anastasia was the wild, free-spirit who later became the hated black sheep in the family. (Photo by Matzene, Butte, Montana, 1917)

Anastasia was now the mistress of Major Victoriano Casajus, the Spanish Military Attaché stationed in Washington as the personal representative of the king and queen of Spain. His wife thought America was an uncivilized place and had chosen to remain back home in Spain with their children. Mary Ellen Kane, the great granddaughter of my grandfather's older half-brother John Patrick, sent me some clippings from her family's collection. One of the clippings from a Washington newspaper mentioned a New Year's Eve dinner dance at the Wardman Park Hotel in 1927. Among the guests were Anastasia and her military attaché, as well as "Miss Eileen O'Meara and Mr. J.W. Carroll." I have no idea who he was, but I hope he was close to my mother's age. Another clipping showed a photo of Major Casajus presenting a model of Christopher Columbus' ship the Santa *Maria* to President Calvin Coolidge. Among the major's charms were invitations to parties at the White House that Anastasia enjoyed immensely. She must have had a particular affinity for distinguished-looking men in uniform because one of the gentlemen in her circle of friends was General Georges Dumont, the French Military Attaché. The mustachioed general and my seventeen-year-old mother struck up an improbable friendship over their shared love of dancing.

It's entirely possible the general didn't know that my mother was only seventeen or it's also possible, but highly unlikely, that his interest in her was purely platonic and he wanted only to learn the latest dances that a girl her age would know much better than his staid contemporaries would. Anastasia's motive, however, was finding an advantageous match for her ward, freeing her of the burdensome responsibility of providing for her sister so she was thrilled when General Dumont began inviting my mother to lunch at his apartment in the Wardman Park Hotel. After the meal, the general would roll up the rug, put records on the phonograph and they would dance vigorously around the room doing the Peabody, the Black Bottom, Charleston and other jazz age dances from the Roaring Twenties. To my mother, the general looked ancient, but he was probably only in his fifties. If anything else happened during her visits to the Wardman Park, my mother never talked about it. But she adamantly did not to marry any of the men her sister introduced her to which angered Anastasia and made her vindictive.

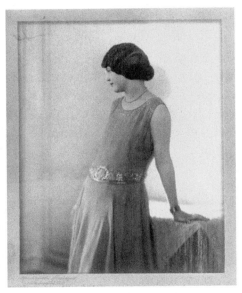

Eileen at the age of 17. On weekends, Anastasia took her little sister out of the convent and introduced her to gentlemen in her sophisticated circle of friends, all of whom were old enough to be Eileen's father. (Photo by Underwood & Underwood, Washington, D.C.)

The nuns were strict, but kind, and my mother thrived in the gentle, serene world of the convent. Ironically, she loved the nuns but not the tenets of Catholicism. Not wanting to shock the nuns, she kept her rebellious questions about church doctrine to herself and quietly did what was expected of a well-brought-up Catholic girl. It wasn't until ten years later, when she was about to marry my father, that she couldn't ignore the clash between her own views and those of the Church. Her mother and both of her grandmothers had each given birth to at least 8 children. Growing up in Butte, most of her friends had come from very large, often boisterous families, some of which struggled to provide adequately for all of their children. She couldn't accept the Catholic Church's position on birth control so she knew it was time to acknowledge what her family had long ago labeled her "heathen tendencies" and leave the church.

Mark and I had a rather ecumenical upbringing, starting out at the Unitarian Church for our most formative years and then attending the Presbyterian Church for a more traditional Christian education. Never at any time, when we were children, do I recall her telling us what we should believe because I think she knew from her own experience that each person has to go on his or her own lifelong quest for spiritual truth.

Our mother sent us to church so that we could decide for ourselves what we believed, but she had no need for organized religion. In fact, I think she was relieved when Mark and I asked if we could switch from the Unitarian Church in Plainfield where we didn't know anybody to the Presbyterian Church in Metuchen where our friends went because then she could stay home and sleep late while we walked to Sunday school by ourselves. At my Unitarian Sunday school, we had conducted science experiments and Jesus was never mentioned.

At the age of ten, there was a part of me that yearned for the security my friends seemed to feel when they sang

"Jesus loves me, yes I know, for the Bible tells me so." I derived an almost guilty satisfaction in going to summer Bible school with one of my friends where we made collages depicting stories in the Bible like baby Moses being rescued from the bulrushes by Pharaoh's daughter. I say guilty because although I don't recall my mother ever saying I shouldn't go to Bible school, I must have intuitively sensed that she didn't want me lured into an unquestioning faith. At any rate, by the age of 12, when I went through confirmation classes, I knew it was too late. I was too shy to ask questions and I couldn't even begin at that age to articulate my doubts, but when all of us in the class stood up in church to recite the Apostles Creed, I had two fingers crossed behind my back as Dr. Behrenburg officially welcomed us into the Presbyterian Church.

12

When my mother graduated from the convent boarding school at the age of seventeen, she was awarded a partial scholarship to attend college. While her older brother was able to go to college and law school, Anastasia and Mollie ordered my mother back home to Butte because they believed education was wasted on women. They told her that her goal in life should be finding a wealthy husband, something that had, so far, eluded them. Anastasia was still seething over her younger sister's refusal to attach herself to any of the rich, older men she introduced my mother to when she was a student at the convent. After all, Grandma Medin had introduced her nineteen-year-old sister Maggie to Marco's best friend, a man twice her age and the marriage, by all accounts, seemed to have been a happy one. Marrying for money was one of the best options available to women in those days, especially if they were lucky enough to be pretty and could be somewhat choosy. My mother chose instead to bide her time working at Hennessey's Department store in Butte, save her money, and then make her escape.

The three years between high school graduation and her decision to leave Butte were unpleasant ones for my mother. The house on West Granite Street had been sold and she had to live in a small apartment with her brother Harney who was just starting out as a new attorney. My mother never fully explained what happened between her and her siblings, but Anastasia ended up the hated black sheep who tried to steal my mother's share of whatever was left of the estate. Uncle Harney had to initiate a law suit on my mother's behalf once she turned 18 and was no longer Anastasia's ward. By this time, Anastasia was living in Washington, D.C. again but no one in the family apparently knew where because a 1928 letter from my mother asking for her share of the estate was addressed to her sister, in care of Roy P. Leahy in Montana Senator Burton K. Wheeler's D.C. office.

By 1932, Anastasia must have fallen on hard times because she had been locked out of her apartment at either the Hotel Harrington or the Hotel Grafton for not paying her bill and most of her possessions that were still in her room had been confiscated and put up for auction, including Grandma Medin's coral necklace and matching broach that had been made by the Italian artist Benvenuto Cellini. Marco and Sarah had bought them in an antique jewelry store in Naples during one of their trips to Europe.

Uncle Harney initiated a law suit on my mother's behalf to get back my mother's share of the estate that Anastasia had kept for herself. The suit included an itemized list of stocks in various mining companies and local Montana businesses as well as other jewelry that had belonged to their mother and grandmother. Grandma Medin's gold cuff bracelet, a ring with one center diamond surrounded by 8 smaller ones, and a rather rustic-looking diamond pin were recovered, but the coral necklace and broach, the most valuable pieces, were lost forever.

Anastasia was also arrested twice for writing bad checks. The first time, she was able to post bail but didn't show up for her trial. The second time, her bail was $5,000 and no one, not even a professional bondsman would post it. A lurid headline on page 2 of the *Los Angeles Examiner* screamed, **"Girl Unable to Get Bail for Freedom"** with a sidebar over a large photo of her that said, *"Disowned by Family – Anastasia Sarah O'Meara, former convent girl and daughter of aristocratic family, held in prison accused of passing worthless checks after death of father and cessation of regular remittances."*

Under the subheading *"Outcast by Family,"* the article went on to say, *"A sister, when asked to help Anastasia out of her difficulties, replied by letter: Anastasia has not dealt fairly with us, and I would not move to save her from jail if I could. The only word I want to hear of her is that she is dead."* Those words could only have been Mollie's. My mother would have been too reserved to write such a caustic reply, but Mollie and Anastasia had a long-standing antipathy toward each other.

During Anastasia's trial, she used her beauty and copious tears to convince the judge that she just didn't quite understand how checking accounts are supposed to work. She was acquitted and eventually ended up in California where a family acquaintance reported that Anastasia had finally found what she was looking for – a rich husband.

The tragic deaths of her parents and sister in 1918, followed by the bitter feud between her siblings and the ensuing lawsuit over the inheritance were fodder for the town gossips and my mother felt that people were gloating over the downfall of the O'Mearas, making her feel self-conscious and miserable. That sense of people's cruel curiosity when they saw her working in the grocery department of Hennessey's, coupled with the long and bitterly cold winters - sometimes it was 40 below zero - made her eager to leave as soon as possible.

Aunt Mollie had loved her time in New York and supported my mother's desire to move there. She contacted her friends Fred and Rosalba Laist, originally from Montana, to ask them to look after my mother which they were glad to do. Mrs. Laist advised my mother about job prospects at the recently opened New York Hospital and was such a warm, nurturing figure in her life that my mother loved her like a daughter. In those days, young people didn't call adults by their first names and yet calling her "Mrs. Laist" began to feel much too formal so my mother began affectionately calling Rosalba "Mrs. Mommy."

The Laists hosted my parents' wedding in their elegant Fifth Avenue apartment, and when my father suggested a honeymoon visiting his parents in Montana, a horrified Mrs. Mommy gave them a two-week trip to Bermuda instead. By the time my mother was pregnant with Mark, it was Mrs. Mommy who took her shopping for nursery furniture and baby clothes. Fred and Rosalba became my brother's god parents, but soon after Mark was born, Rosalba died suddenly from a congenital heart ailment.

That's how I ended up being named Rosalba. My mother loved Mrs. Laist so much, she wanted to honor her memory in the most fitting way she knew how, but she and my father didn't really like the name. I was christened Rosalba O'Meara Christensen, but was always called Meara except when we were visiting Uncle Fred or his children, a confusing subterfuge which always caused a profound sense of guilt for my brother and me when we were little. One of Mrs. Laist's granddaughters was also named Rosalba, but her family openly called her Robin and even Uncle Fred had called his wife by an affectionate nickname instead of Rosalba so I couldn't understand why I had to be burdened with a name everyone seemed to hate when we were visiting Uncle Fred.

Maybe because Uncle Fred's two daughters Ginny and Dorie were living out in California, he kept up the close relationship with my mother and Mark and me. That first Christmas after my father died in 1947, he sent a limousine out to Metuchen to bring us through a pounding snow storm to spend the holiday with his family in New York. Over the years, we would take the train to New York and the Fifth Avenue bus, back when Fifth Ave. was still a two-way street, up to his elegant apartment overlooking the Central Park reservoir. The uniformed doorman would greet us and a quick ride up in the elevator would bring us to Uncle Fred's rarified world where the grand piano took up just one little corner of the large living room, every room had a working fireplace, even the bedrooms, each of which also had its own bathroom, and servants circulated among the guests passing out hors d'oeuvres. The floors were covered with thick Oriental rugs and an old grandfather clock in the entrance hall chimed on the hour and half-hour.

When Uncle Fred's son Jim and his wife Mildred from Upper Montclair were there with their three children, Mark and I had kids our own age to play with. When they weren't there, Mark and I could sit at the big table with the adults, as long as we listened quietly and didn't speak unless one of the adults specifically asked one of us a question, usually something about school or what we had done in the city that day before arriving at Uncle Fred's apartment. As I sat there trying to be polite and unobtrusive, all I really wanted to do was play with the miniature silver salt cellar with its tiny mother of pearl spoon situated right in front of me. In fact, each guest had an identical salt cellar, but I seemed to be the only one struggling not to play with it. As each course was finished, Uncle Fred's Irish maid Maude and her assistant would miraculously appear from the kitchen with the next dish to be served. Only later did we discover the secret button at the head of the table that Uncle Fred used to summon the maids with the next course.

Sometimes before going to Uncle Fred's our mother would take us ice skating at Rockefeller Center where I could wear my red velveteen skating skirt and pretend I was Sonja Henie, the Norwegian three-time Olympic gold medal winner and movie actress who starred in old films I had seen on television. Other times, she took us to see a show at Radio City Music Hall, where like millions of other little girls, I dreamed of becoming a Rockette when I grew up, or we'd visit the Metropolitan Museum of Art which was just a few blocks south of Uncle Fred's or the Haydn Planetarium on the other side of Central Park.

Mom loved New York and enjoyed introducing us to its cultural advantages. She must have saved up for months to take us to see "Peter Pan" on Broadway, starring Mary Martin. I was still young enough to believe that Peter, Wendy, John and Michael were magically flying and that a real crocodile was crawling across the stage in pursuit of Captain Hook. Standing in front of my seat in the balcony for a better view, I held my breath waiting to see what would be his fate. Many years later, when Dana and Jay were little, Mom treated us all to the Broadway revival of "Peter Pan," starring Sandy Duncan.

Back in the early 1950's, when we traveled into New York on the Pennsylvania Railroad, we rode on some of the last trains still pulled by steam locomotives. After a sometimes terrifying ride through the old tunnel under the Hudson River, when the train would often stall for some unexplained reason and sparks would rain down on us, still with no explanation from the conductors, we would eventually arrive at Penn Station, the grand Beaux Arts building built in 1911 that looked like a magnificent Greek temple. The station in Metuchen where we left from was a one-room red wooden structure fitting for a small town, but the old Penn Station in New York inspired awe. Clutching my mother's hand, as her high heels clicked smartly on the marble floor, I would gaze up at the enormous Corinthian columns lining the interior of the great hall and gape in amazement. This was the appropriate way to enter one of the greatest cities in the world and I was suitably impressed.

By 1964, when I was attending art school in New York, the city was in the process of tearing down this magnificent structure in order to sell the air space above the train tracks to the latest incarnation of Madison Square Garden. Each morning, when we arrived in the city, commuters had to negotiate a new labyrinth of detours in order to find our way out of the building, only to deal with a new set of detours when we returned at the end of the day. The end result was a monstrosity that is destined for the wrecking ball in the twenty-first century. While riding into the city every morning from 1964 to 1967, crossing the Jersey Meadowlands, I watched New York's famous skyline be transformed as the Twin Towers of the World Trade Center were being built. Completed in 1971, the towers were the tallest buildings in the world for a time, only to be tragically destroyed by terrorists on the morning of September 11, 2001.

Jay was 26 and working in the financial district in lower Manhattan. Dana was an editor at Wine Spectator Magazine in mid-town New York. I had just arrived at my job at the Community FoodBank of New Jersey when a co-worker talking to someone on the phone yelled, "A plane just crashed into the World Trade Center!" Everyone quickly assumed that it had to have been a horrible, freakish accident because no civilized human being would do such a thing on purpose. I ran upstairs to my boss's office where the only television in the building was located. Co-workers gathered around the small TV and watched in horror as, a few moments later, news cameras showed a second plane flying into the other tower. Newscasters reported another plane had flown into the Pentagon and a fourth hijacked plane was in the air somewhere over Pennsylvania.

The country was under attack, but no one knew the full extent yet as the government scrambled to respond. I knew that Jay traveled into New York via the PATH train that passed under the World Train Center and watched in horror as this tragedy unfolded. Meanwhile, Dana and Carlos could see it all from their living room window in Weehawken. She was just about to leave for the city when the first plane hit the tower and stayed where she was because all tunnels under the Hudson were immediately closed. After an interminable wait, my phone rang and it was Jay telling me that he was safe. Right after that, it was almost impossible to reach anyone by phone because the cell towers on top of the World Trade Center were destroyed and all other communications lines were overloaded.

Jay had passed through the World Trade Center PATH station just 15 minutes before the first plane hit and his office building 4 blocks away was locked down to prevent anyone from entering or leaving because all the surrounding streets were clogged with smoke and falling debris and trapped vehicles that had nowhere to flee. From Jay's building, they could see desperate people jumping from the burning towers, a nightmarish image that was singed into memories forever.

My mother, fortunately, was blissfully ignorant of all this.

13

After two years at Rose Hall, the time came when I had to move my mother over to the Special Care Unit and discontinue the services of Ivy, the live-in aide I had hired to give my mother the close attention she needed, because the monthly fee for her apartment and the cost of a live-in aide were $8,000 a month. My mother was living longer than she or I had expected and now some painful choices had to be made.

When my mother's dementia had made it necessary to move her to assisted living, I made the decision without a qualm because I knew it was best for her safety. But when I had to fire the aide, who had lived with and cared for my mother for two years, I suddenly felt the need to join an Alzheimer's support group to explore these new feelings of uncertainly and depression about whether I was doing the right thing. The part that depressed me was the knowledge that I wasn't doing what was best for my mother's sense of security and peace of mind. It was just an economic necessity because, although her dementia was getting worse, her heart was strong and she could live to be 100.

To ease my mother's transition in the new location I kept Ivy on for a week. On her first morning without her familiar caretaker, I took time off from work and went to visit her. I found her sitting on a bench in the hallway outside her new room. She didn't know where she belonged and kept repeating over and over that everything dear to her had been taken away. I sat down on the bench and put my arm around her as we both cried.

Ivy, fortunately, had been assigned to a new case at Rose Hall and she came to see my mother for a brief visit each day. By this time, my mother's memory stopped somewhere back in her early childhood and she thought Ivy had been her nurse when she was little. When my mother was difficult and uncooperative, the aides in Special Care would call Ivy to help coax her through her bad moods.

As my mother became more child-like, we found new ways to reach her through child-like pleasures – she loved picture books, especially stories about animals and happy families. Birthdays and Christmases became occasions to give colorful storybooks and teddy bears. On Mother's Day, I gave her a small brown bear with just the right hopeful expression in its shiny black eyes. I had gone to at least half-a-dozen stores interviewing a multitude of teddy bears until I had found the one with the right softness and appealing facial expression, and when I gave it to her, it was love at first sight. The bear became her best friend and confidant and accompanied her everywhere in the saddle bag attached to her walker.

Her favorite outing was a trip to the park to feed the ducks. In the beginning, she'd walk down the path to the lake; later, I'd wheel her in a borrowed wheel chair with the bag of cracked corn clutched firmly in her lap. I'd look around for an isolated spot and pretend I didn't see the sign warning people that feeding the water fowl was strictly prohibited.

She'd toss out a handful of corn and wait hopefully. Unaccustomed to being fed by humans, it usually took a few minutes before she was surrounded by Canada geese, ducks and pigeons. More than anything, she loved having them eat out of her hand, and when a beautiful swan trusted her enough to reach its long neck out and delicately eat the corn she offered, my mother beamed with unequivocal delight. I captured that moment on film and shared it with the rest of the family.

Eventually, the park's department put up more warning signs than I could pretend not to see so we shifted to indoor strolls up and down the aisles of Target and Kohl's where we were sure to see some mothers wheeling their babies who fascinated her just as much as ducks and swans did.

Another favorite destination was Barnes & Noble. Her love of books was so much a part of her being that she enjoyed wandering past the shelves just soaking in the sight and smell of them. One day she said, "If I had the money, I'd buy them all!" without remembering that she once had owned thousands of books. Every room but the bathroom in her house in Metuchen had contained shelves filled with books on every subject imaginable. Even when her cataracts and, later, her failing memory made it difficult to read with pleasure she still kept buying books.

When she was a child, her parents' house had one room that was designated "the library," filled with leather-bound volumes of Dickens, Balzac, Jane Austen, the Brontë sisters and other classics, as well as popular children's literature. Being the youngest of eight children with an eight-year gap between her and her brother Harney and an eighteen-year gap between her and her oldest sister

Anastasia, my mother must have felt at times like an only child with no one to play with at home. Books became her most sought-after companions and this affinity lasted her entire life.

Because she had, at a very young age, taught herself how to read, she assumed that I would be equally eager to learn. When, in first grade, I was placed in the second reading group, the look on her face was unmistakable. I suppose most mothers have the power to convey to their children exactly what they're thinking simply by raising or lowering an eyebrow or adjusting the turn of their lips, but my mother always had a distressingly open countenance. I knew I was in trouble. The teacher's notation on my report card indicated I lacked enthusiasm for books and preferred drawing instead, prompting my mother to sit me down at my little table, the one where I liked having tea parties, and presented me with a pile of children's books to study. They all had a daunting number of words on each page and only a smattering of small, uninspiring line drawings.

I was miserable at being tortured this way. In school, we were forced to read nonsense like, "Look, Alice, look! See Gip run! Run, Gip, run." This drivel went on for pages and pages and as a further irritation, Alice and her friend May always wore dresses when they played outside and the illustrations showed them standing passively, with their hands behind their backs, watching Jerry play with a ball or climb trees. I had concluded early in the school year that if this is what reading is all about, I didn't want to be bothered. But by second grade, we were presented with a whole new group of more interesting characters who had real adventures and I was hooked. My mother was pleased when I was placed in the first reading group and I was ready to be introduced to the *Wizard of Oz* series, *The Little Colonel*, *Anne of Green Gables* and some of her other favorite books from childhood.

Some mothers fit the 1950's style of gentle, pampering nurturer made popular in TV sitcoms, but my mother was more of a stern, no nonsense nurturer. Mark and I knew she loved us, but as soon as she deemed we were old enough, she expected us to pitch in and do our share of the work. While she went to the doctor's office to work on Saturday mornings, we were supposed to clean the house. At the ages of six and ten, I don't suppose we had the attention span to really apply ourselves and do a good job. In between sweeping, dusting and emptying the waste baskets, we spent most of our time playing while listening to Martin Block's "Make Believe Ballroom" until we heard the old DeSoto pull into the driveway and our hearts started to pound. Luckily for us, she wasn't a finicky housekeeper so our distracted efforts were generally passable enough.

By the time I was ten, we got our first television, creating an even bigger distraction on Saturday mornings. Rocky and Bullwinkle, Crusader Rabbit, Boris and Natasha, Dudley Do-Right and the Fractured Fairytales kept us mesmerized until the spell was broken by the DeSoto's motor purring in the driveway and Mark rushed upstairs to pretend he was cleaning his room, leaving me with a sink full of dishes soaking in cold, greasy water.

At an early age, Mark expressed an interest in becoming an architect when he grew up so our mother was eager to encourage him. Before long, our backyard was a little shanty town of forts that Mark designed and proudly built from a random assortment of old shutters and cast off screens from our house combined with scrap lumber that he had pilfered from several building sites up the street where new houses were being constructed in the former woods. He even built a fort high up in a huge sycamore tree in the yard behind ours until the neighbors, concerned that he might fall to his death, demanded that he take it down. Looking back on it now, I wonder if old Mrs. Carmen on one side of us and the Everetts on the other side ever complained about the view from their windows.

When my mother's boss bought a new car in 1956, she bought his pea green Packard from him and the old DeSoto went up on cinder blocks in the back yard waiting until Mark was old enough to drive it.

On the back pages of Mark's comic books, there were always ads for get rich quick schemes for entrepreneurial little kids who were willing to go door-to-door selling things. First he sold wrapping paper, then greeting cards and candy, before moving on to handy household gadgets that might appeal to housewives. The most useful item was a small fire extinguisher, the kind of thing that every family should have in the kitchen. Mark created his own clever marketing strategy that involved a metal wastebasket and a wad of newspapers. He'd place the waste basket on a neighbor's front porch, set the papers on fire and then ring the doorbell. When the startled housewife opened her door and screamed, he'd step forward and put the fire out. Some of the women were impressed by his ingenuity and bought a fire extinguisher while others were shaking with rage and called my mother to complain. I don't know how many he sold, but years later, I would come across these tiny extinguishers in the backs of drawers and in boxes down in the basement, along with left over wrapping paper samples and greeting cards. Eventually, he got a paper route selling *The Perth Amboy Evening News* after school, until he was old enough to get his working papers and a job at Metuchen Center selling toys and sporting goods. Half his pay went into his college fund and the rest was spent on model airplane kits, Mad Magazine and rock 'n roll records.

14

When I was young, my mother subscribed to a daily newspaper, but I don't recall seeing her do more than glance at the headlines and peruse the lead paragraphs of a few articles. I think sometimes the outside world and all its many problems were more than she wanted to have to think about when she had enough worries of her own. In my early teens, I wasn't much interested in the international turmoil and domestic political skullduggery either. Except for when a teacher gave the class a current events report, I never read anything in the paper beyond Anne Landers' advice column and the comics.

The ever-present Cold War tensions between the United States and the Soviet Union were always lurking in the background creating a helpless sense of fear that was too painful to dwell on. When a company selling backyard bomb shelters set up a display on Main Street in the mid 1950's, my mother toyed briefly with the idea of buying one until she decided it would be better not to survive a nuclear holocaust. She compromised by having shelves built in the basement and stocking them with hundreds of cans of vegetables, soup, Beefaroni, tuna, and her favorite, deviled ham. Every so often, bulging cans had to be discarded and replaced with a new supply – just in case.

The saying of the day was, "Better dead than red!" When that slogan was posted on a bulletin board in my high school, I remember thinking, "But if everyone who is opposed to communism chooses death, who will be around to restore democratic capitalism when people begin to realize that communism is contrary to human nature?" Early on, I decided that communism wasn't the thing we should fear, but rather nuclear annihilation over a dispute about differing, and ultimately temporary, political systems. Since the beginning of recorded time, political systems have come and gone, but Earth is the only planet we have and nothing could ever be worth destroying it.

The Bay of Pigs Invasion early in President John Kennedy's term in office, followed in 1962 by the Cuban Missile Crisis began to shatter the wall of willful apathy in which my mother and I had enclosed ourselves. The situation in far-away Vietnam began occupying more space in the newspapers as the United States' increasing involvement with that country's internal problems became apparent. After the corrupt President Ngo Dinh Diem was assassinated on November 2, with help from the CIA in the 1963 coup, and President Kennedy was assassinated just twenty days later, shaking the confidence of the entire country, the world seemed out of control.

Before long, the newspapers were filled with reports about the growing "Vietnam crisis" and the urgent rumblings in Congress about the need to stop the spread of communism in Southeast Asia. Despite my ambiguous religious training, I began praying nightly, and at random intervals throughout the day, that God wouldn't allow this "crisis" to turn into all-out war. Young men were being drafted and Mark, as well as all the boys I ever knew, were at the vulnerable target age.

By this time, Mark was working full-time and putting himself through college. After one semester at Rensselaer Polytechnic Institute where he had planned to study architecture, Mark changed his mind and came home. Somewhere between his childhood dream of building things and his classes at RPI in advanced calculus and trigonometry, he realized he really wanted to be a journalist. Our mother was not pleased about his dropping out of school and hitchhiking home in the middle of winter. Her disappointment in him, coupled with her impatience at what she perceived to be his mule-headed stubbornness, led to Mark's decision to move out on his own, requiring him to work full-time to support himself. If he had remained at home and commuted to college, as she wanted, he could have gone to school full-time, but he was intent on being independent.

Mark transferred to Fairleigh Dickenson in Rutherford, New Jersey, and became very active with the American Civil Liberties Union. He almost single-handedly wrote and edited the ACLU newspaper on campus and was following the crisis in Vietnam very closely because anti-communist paranoia was beginning to squelch public criticism of our rapidly escalating military involvement in defense of a corrupt right-wing dictatorship that didn't even have the support of the South Vietnamese people.

Lyndon Johnson had won the 1964 presidential election in a landslide against Barry Goldwater, largely because he wasn't perceived to be a warmonger like Goldwater who had suggested it might be necessary to use tactical nuclear weapons against North Vietnam.

Nevertheless, more and more young men were being sent to Vietnam to prop up the South Vietnamese government whose only claim to legitimacy was that it was anti-communist. I worried constantly about Mark and my boyfriend at the time being drafted.

From once avoiding the news, I now couldn't get enough. Mark introduced me to all the progressive publications he read like *Ramparts, The New Republic, Mother Jones,* and of course, *The New York Times.* He also gave me David Halberstam's *The Making of a Quagmire,* the Pulitzer Prize-winning book tracing the growth of U.S. involvement in Vietnam.

By 1965, I was in my second year of art school at the New York-Phoenix School of Design and was taking night classes at Rutgers in New Brunswick. For my freshman English term paper, I wrote about the growing student protest movement against the war in Vietnam. For an essay assignment based on Jonathan Swift's *A Modest Proposal,* I wrote that young men should be spared and only the old men should be drafted to fight wars because it's always old men who start them. If all countries adopted this policy, wars would be over quickly because most old men wouldn't survive basic training, let alone the hardship of battle. The essay was satirical, of course, but there was a part of me that longed for it to be true.

I can trace this part of my life as the transition from willful apathy to a perpetual state of righteous indignation, mentally arguing with people who mindlessly accepted whatever the government did despite the impossibility of winning a war in support of a government that was just as cruel and repressive as any communist regime. Opposition candidates in Vietnam were jailed and people were shot in the street simply for being suspected of being Vietcong agents. Everyone knew that Vietnamese President Nguyen Cao Ký and Vice President Nguyen Van Thieu just kept trading places in a series of rigged elections, while Buddhist monks in Vietnam publically immolated themselves in protest. I became almost dizzy with rage when fellow students would say things like, "President Johnson must be right or he wouldn't be president." My boyfriend at the time, a Rutgers junior comfortably safe with his college deferment, told me that "war is good because it's good for the economy."

Early in 1966, the thing my mother and I feared most happened: Mark received his 1A notice from his draft board. Despite working full-time and taking 12 credits a semester, just three credits short of a full-time student, and despite being on the dean's list, his draft board concluded that he wasn't really a serious student and therefore not eligible for a deferment. For some reason, Mark chose not to contest the decision, nor would he leave for Canada as thousands of young men were doing. He declined my rather reckless, but very earnest, offer to permanently maim him somehow so he'd fail his physical and instead paid a visit to the enlistment offices of each branch of the military to see which one could offer him a position that didn't involve killing people in exchange for offering himself up for a 3-year commitment.

When I angrily told him I didn't believe there was anything dishonorable in dodging this particular war, he said he worried about what pro-war zealots might do to my mother and me. In 1966, the majority of Americans still accepted the domino theory of communist paranoia, people who avoided the draft could be arrested, and violent street fights regularly broke out when anti-war activists dared to protest in public.

For this reason, my mother was very uneasy when I went to New York for the first march and mass rally against the Vietnam War, but she didn't try to talk me out of going. None of my friends would go with me, not even my boyfriend, so I took the train into the city by myself. As a concession to my mother, I skipped the march down Fifth Avenue where I learned later that some people had actually been punched or pelted with rocks, and headed directly for the rally in front of the United Nations.

By some estimates, more than 300,000 people were jammed onto First Avenue, FDR Drive and all the side streets leading up to the stage in front of the United Nations where speaker after speaker called for an end to our involvement in Vietnam's civil war. Demonstrations and rallies against the war were happening in major cities and college campuses all over the country, but it made no difference to the Johnson administration.

Mark ultimately chose to go into the Army because they offered him a position in the Intelligence Corp where he'd be sitting at a desk in Saigon instead of carrying a gun through the jungle looking for people to kill. Before reporting for basic training at Fort Dix in South Jersey, he worked on bulking up his thin frame through strenuous exercise combined with doubling his caloric intake.

Meanwhile, a nineteen-year-old private who had just reported to Fort Dix a few weeks before Mark was due to leave home, died from pneumonia at Walson Army Hospital. His name was Andrew and he had just married his high school sweetheart before going off to war. Andrew had caught the flu during basic training and was admitted to the base hospital where he complained that he couldn't breathe. But instead of giving him oxygen, the army nurses told him to stop complaining and just get up and walk around to clear his lungs. The next day he was found dead. The newspaper said there would be an investigation.

My mother carried on stoically in the weeks leading up to Mark's departure, but I knew she feared the worst because she sent him to a photographer to have a formal portrait done. She didn't say she wanted something to remember him by, of course, but Mark and I knew.

Shortly after Mark reported for basic training, he became sick and was sent to Walson Army Hospital. My mother and I drove down to see him but when we got to his ward, he wasn't in his assigned bed or anywhere in sight. We anxiously wandered around looking for someone to ask when he suddenly walked out of the men's room carrying a mop and bucket. I don't know if treating all hospital patients as though they are lying malingerers is a standard procedure in the army or if Walson was a particularly bad example, but it served to fuel my anger and mistrust of the military. I vented my anger by writing letters to every member of Congress who had ever said anything indicating they had doubts about our involvement in Vietnam. I was becoming obsessed.

Sometimes I wonder how Mark calmly handled being coerced into postponing his education and going off to assist in a war he didn't support while I was filled with impotent rage. I got into arguments with classmates and even strangers who believed the war was necessary and could be reduced to tears when I thought of all the young men who were dying before they even had a chance to fulfill any of their aspirations.

During this period, I happened to go to a dance at Rutgers with a friend of mine on April 15, 1966. I remember the date because that's the night I met Bruce, the man who became my husband. I had been having very conflicted feelings about Harry, the boy I had been dating for the past two years. He's the one who thought war was good because it's good for the economy, and he ridiculed the American Civil Liberties Union, a forty-six year-old organization I had recently joined, calling it a "fly-by-night" group that was probably engaged in all kinds of nefarious activities. He was especially scornful of the anti-war movement. On the one hand, he was sexy and fun to be with, and he drove a convertible, something young women, even one as serious as I was, found attractive. But one night, as we drove home from the Asbury Park boardwalk, he shouted a racist epithet to a group of black teenagers and he often referred to other ethnic groups as "kikes," "spics," or "dagos." I criticized his racist behavior, but he just thought it was funny. Then, one night when he said he wanted to be able to go out with other girls occasionally, I said, "Good idea; you do that. And I'll be free to go out with other boys." It was time to move on.

That was undoubtedly the best decision I ever made in my life because I was standing there at the edge of the dance floor, unencumbered by Harry, when a sophomore named Bruce walked up and asked me to dance. After we danced a while, we decided to sit down and talk which led inevitably, at least for me at that stage in my life, to a discussion of the war. At that time, he was still a believer in the domino theory that if we let Vietnam fall to communism, soon all of Southeast Asia would be communist, but at least his feelings were earnestly based on principle, not crass war profiteering and he had some good points to make. He wasn't just being stupidly flippant and dismissive, like Harry. When he told me he was a member of the campus chapter of the NAACP, I was impressed and was glad when he asked for my phone number.

For the first two years of our courtship, we went for walks and picnics, visited museums, saw lots of movies, went to dances at Rutgers and spent a great deal of time arguing about the war. My intensity of feeling would have driven a lesser man away, but Bruce liked that I was different from the other girls he had dated. However, at one point in the spring of 1967, my temper flared more than usual and we actually broke up over the war. But that weekend, when Bruce's mother Jean died suddenly of a pulmonary embolism, I rushed to be with him and our argument was forgotten.

A few weeks later, a friend of Bruce's father gave him four box seat tickets to a NY Yankees game, but he didn't feel like going to a baseball game so soon after his wife's death so he gave the tickets to Bruce and his brother Michael and his first wife Barbara. We were sitting right behind first base when Mickey Mantle hit a home run in the bottom of the ninth inning to win the game against the Minnesota Twins. Even I thought it was exciting, but Bruce, who was a lifelong Yankees fan, was ecstatic.

Later that night, we were sitting in his car talking in front of my mother's house. I had just graduated from art school and was planning to save my salary from my first job as a commercial artist so that I could spend the following summer touring Europe. Some of my friends from school were also planning to save their money so we could all travel together, but I didn't have much confidence that they were as committed as I was. I told Bruce that it would really be much more fun to travel with him, but he reminded me that my mother would *not* approve. I said, "She wouldn't mind, if we were married." I don't believe women should be passive when it comes to important decisions in life, but at that time in my life

I wouldn't have had the nerve to propose if we hadn't already talked about getting married someday.

We decided to officially get engaged at Christmas, but I kept putting off telling my mother about our plans. She liked Bruce, but she had decided opinions about an appropriate age for marriage and I knew she would think 22 was much too young. She also was suspicious of Catholics because of the church's opposition to birth control, so the fact that Bruce had been raised Catholic was a big black mark against him, despite the fact that he was non-practicing and hadn't been to church in years, except for funerals and weddings. But my biggest concern was how she would face the sudden realization that when I married, she would be alone.

By this time, Mark was about half-way through his tour in Vietnam so I decided to wait until he was safely home before telling her. At least that would alleviate some of her anxiety. Bruce was due to graduate from Rutgers the following June so we figured we could set a date once we knew if he'd be drafted.

15

Each generation is tested in some way: our parents had the Great Depression and World War II that led to them being labeled "the greatest generation." Our grandparents and great grandparents faced wars, famine, religious persecution, economic stagnation – any number of problems that had to be overcome which helped lead to the settling of America.

But the kids born during the Baby Boom generation spent their childhoods with the threat of nuclear annihilation, coupled with the need to recognize and subsequently change how we and our parents' generation treated African Americans. What should have been a civilized and peaceful adjustment in a country that prides itself on its exemplary family values, often turned out to be marred by hatred and violence.

Throughout the fifties and sixties, our sensibilities were assaulted by images on the nightly news of black men in suits and ties, women and children, dressed as if on their way to church, being chased by club-wielding police on horseback. People simply trying to register to vote or enjoy the same privileges granted to whites in the Bill of Rights led to their being sprayed with tear gas, attacked by vicious police dogs or even killed in assassinations or lynchings. Four young girls were murdered and twenty others injured during Sunday school when the Ku Klux Klan bombed the 16th Street Baptist Church in

Birmingham, Alabama. Civil rights workers, including white volunteers from up north, were beaten and even murdered for trying to desegregate the south.

White people's complacency was being shattered and a more enlightened way of looking at race relations slowly, and often reluctantly, evolved. During the long, hot summer of 1967, 125 American cities erupted in violence. One of the most destructive uprisings occurred in Newark, New Jersey, the city where I was working after graduation from art school.

That June, I was hired as a display designer at Hahne and Company, an upscale department store on Broad Street. African Americans in Newark were clustered in one of the nation's poorest ghettos, and according to a documentary on PBS, the city also had the nation's highest percentage of substandard housing, and the second highest rates of crime and infant mortality. With this volatile mixture, a reported case of police brutality against a black cab driver one night in July plunged the city into five days of violence in which 26 people died, 1,100 people were injured and fires and looting resulted in more than $10 million in damages.

From the relative safety of the store, my co-workers and I watched smoke rising in the sky as neighborhoods a few blocks away burned and National Guardsmen and state troopers were called in to cordon off parts of the city to try to quell the riots. Sniper fire was reported in many parts of the city and machine guns could be heard in downtown Newark. Through all this, the store remained open, although very few people were venturing into Newark to shop. For those of us who commuted to work by train, the personnel department thought it would be a wise move to assign each of their employees a buddy for the walk to the train station at night, and I was matched with a woman who liked taking short cuts through deserted parking lots on her way back to Penn Station. I preferred walking out on the street with other pedestrians so she and I went our separate ways. Through it all, I never heard of any white pedestrians being accosted by the black residents of Newark. Their anger seemed to be concentrated against law enforcement and businesses in predominantly black neighborhoods, which sadly, ultimately hurt the people who already were suffering.

I don't think my mother and I realized at the time just how bad the riots were. I know we hadn't read that President Johnson had contacted New Jersey's Governor Hughes offering to send federal troops, but Mark, almost 9,000 miles away in the middle of the war in Vietnam, was reading all the fearsome details and was very worried about my safety here in New Jersey!

The riots ended and a fretful calm settled over the smoldering city. On the nights that I had to work until 9:00 p.m., Bruce drove into Newark and picked me up outside the employee entrance so I wouldn't have to walk through the city alone.

In the tumultuous spring of 1968, civil rights leader Dr. Martin Luther King, Jr. was assassinated in Memphis and just two months later, Robert Kennedy was gunned down after winning the Democratic primary in California. In that unsettled environment, Bruce graduated from Rutgers with the threat of the draft hanging over our plans for the future. When we had first met, he had intended to go to law school after graduation, but the recent riots and the civil rights movement made him reevaluate his goal for an eventual career in politics. Teaching in the Newark school system or social work became decidedly more relevant for an idealistic young man like him, coupled with our ardent hope that his draft board might think helping poor people in Newark was more important than killing Vietnamese peasants.

By September of that year, Bruce had found a job doing social work in some of Newark's most dangerous neighborhoods. At that time, caseworkers visited welfare clients in their apartments where they were sometimes threatened on the streets by gang members and drug dealers. Most of the time, though, residents knew if they saw a white person walking in the neighborhood, more often than not, it was a welfare worker so they were usually left alone.

In October, Bruce's father Michael suffered a sudden heart attack and died after a short hospital stay. It was seventeen months after Bruce's mother Jean had died, but his father had never gotten over the loss of his beloved wife. They had been through so many hardships – Jean was hit by a car soon after their marriage and suffered back problems for the rest of her life, their first-born child, and only daughter, was stillborn; when their three sons were very young, Michael developed colon cancer and had a colostomy; and Jean became diabetic with all the other health risks that diabetes entails. The doctors thought Michael was sterile because of his cancer treatments, but rather miraculously, and to the family's great surprise, Bruce was conceived and born on September 22, 1946.

Michael and Jean had put four boys through college, three of them at the same time, and were finally at a stage in life when they could slow down and enjoy themselves. They planned to travel, and in fact, had been packed and ready to go on a trip when she died suddenly the night before. Bruce believes to this day that his father was just waiting for him to get a job so he could take care of himself and then his father would be free to die of a broken heart.

Throughout that fall and winter, there was no word from Bruce's draft board so we dared to go ahead and plan our wedding for May of 1969. With both of his parents so recently deceased, it seemed most appropriate to have a small, simple wedding rather than a lavish formal dinner as was rapidly becoming the trend among couples our age. We got married in the Church of the Little Flower, the Catholic Church in Berkeley Heights where his family had gone, because Bruce seemed concerned that if we married in a Protestant Church, his Aunt Millie would think we were living in sin. This, of course, did not please my mother, but since I wasn't at all religious, I didn't feel it mattered much one way or the other. To please my mother, we had Dr. Behrenberg, the minister from the Presbyterian Church in Metuchen, assist Father Arico in performing the ceremony. We had a reception for 75 guests at the Westfield Women's Club which had the feel of a gracious home instead of a commercial catering hall.

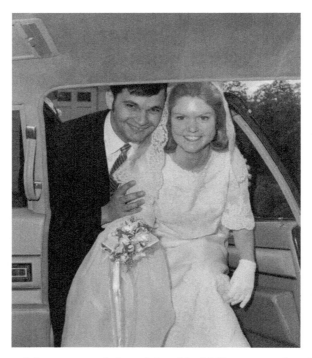

Bruce and I were married on May 10, 1969, two weeks after he received his 1A notice from his draft board. (Photo by Bejas Studios, Woodbridge, NJ)

We spent our first two nights in a bridal suite at New York's Plaza Hotel for the astoundingly low sum of $50, which included champagne and an elegant breakfast served in our private sitting room. Something like that would probably cost more than $500 a night now, if the Plaza were still operating as a hotel. We got the great deal through a coupon I found in *Brides Magazine*. On Sunday morning, we took a romantic handsome cab ride through Central Park and then had dinner at Tavern on the Green. On Monday, we sailed for Europe on The

Nieuw Amsterdam, fulfilling a dream for which I had saved most of my earnings for the past two years.

A small yellow bi-plane followed the ship as we sailed down the Hudson, then dipped its wings as we left the New York skyline behind. Passing under the Verrazano Narrows Bridge and sailing into the open waters of the Atlantic, I felt as though we were making our escape because, with ironic timing, Bruce's 1A notice had finally arrived a few days before our wedding. By law, once he received this notice from his draft board, he was not supposed to leave the country, but we were not going to let the war in Vietnam ruin our plans. We just hoped he wouldn't be called for his physical before we returned home six weeks later.

This amazing honeymoon, consisting of sailing round-trip across the Atlantic, two Eurail Passes for unlimited rail travel within Europe, hotels, breakfasts and tours in each city cost us only $2,000 because we had the cheapest cabin on the ship and booked our hotels through the *Europe on $5 a Day* program. Our tiny windowless cabin on the ship was below the water line, smelled faintly of salt water, had bunk beds and no private bathroom, but we were thrilled beyond words to be crossing the ocean and embarking on a wonderful adventure. It may have been Spartan compared with the first class accommodations on the ship's upper decks, but it was very luxurious compared with the crowded sailing vessel that took six weeks to bring the Thornton family to America in the 1840's, or the steam ship that my grandfather came to American on in 1880. It was even very Spartan compared with the ships we sailed on to Europe and the Caribbean later in our marriage, when passengers had come to expect every amenity and diversion imaginable to enhance the journey.

On the Nieuw Amsterdam, in 1969, however, the morning's highlight was bullion served on deck at 11:00, and we all looked forward with excitement to tea and pastries at 4:00 in the one and only lounge where the same band played dance music every afternoon and evening. Although we were in second class, we all dressed for dinner every night. No shorts and tee shirts on this trip.

We took a northerly route across the Atlantic, following roughly the same route the ill-fated Titanic had taken in the reverse direction in 1912. One day, the sea was so rough, passengers were forbidden to venture out on deck for fear they'd be washed overboard, and most people stayed in bed. Bruce was feeling sea sick, but I need to eat no matter how I feel so I dressed and went up to the main deck to find some food. Very few people were out and about, and those of us who were tired of lying in bed found that we could navigate the open lobby area only by pulling ourselves along on ropes that were stretched from wall to wall. I was one of the only people in the dining room that night, and fortunately, the ocean was much calmer for the rest of the crossing.

After six days at sea, we anchored off the coast of Cobh, Ireland, the port my grandfather most likely sailed from, and tenders brought over the passengers who were disembarking in Ireland, returning with several Irish women who were permitted on board to sell their handmade fisherman-knit sweaters and lace tablecloths. We bought two tablecloths, but the wool sweaters were too itchy and had to be passed by.

The next day, we docked in Southampton, England, and only those passengers booked for the U.K. were allowed off the ship. We stood on deck watching as cargo, including vehicles, were off-loaded.

By the eighth day, we docked in Rotterdam and began our exploration of Europe. Not wanting to activate our Eurail Passes yet, we took a cab all the way to Amsterdam, the first city on our itinerary. Even if we could have afforded to stay in first class hotels, our objective was to experience Europe as average Europeans did so we had chosen second class pensions, which it turned out, were often just a step above youth hostels. Our first hotel, whose name we still remember almost 50 years later, was the Hotel Ardina. We remember it because it was so comically awful it made an indelible impression that time could not erase.

Again, we must have had the cheapest accommodation being offered because our room was up in the attic where we could stand up straight only in the center of the peaked ceiling. There was a 60 watt light bulb in the center of the room, but the electricity went off at 8:00 a.m. and didn't come back on until evening. We had twin beds on opposite ends of the long, narrow room, but we were flexible so we just pushed them together to make it almost as good as a king-size bed. There was a tiny sink against one wall with a mirror mounted above it on the steep ceiling, providing an excellent view of the undersides of our chins. The toilet was on the floor below which could be accessed by climbing down the carpeted ladder that served as the only staircase in the building. Climbing down wasn't so bad, but climbing up when we arrived with our luggage was a challenge. We learned that many years ago, when Amsterdam was being built, taxes were levied on the width of a building, but not the height. Therefore, thrifty Amsterdamers built tall, narrow structures with ladders, or sometimes very steep staircases, between floors.

On May first, most Dutch hotels, or at least the less expensive ones, turn off the heat regardless of the outside temperature and May, 1969, was a particularly chilly spring in Holland. I was very cold and out of desperation had covered my filmy honeymoon nightgown with one of Bruce's sweaters and a pair of his slacks. To complete the picture, my shoulder-length hair was done up in rollers, a torturous affliction that women had to put up with back in the 60's. As I backed down the ladder, two men in the room below started laughing at me. I knew I looked ridiculous so all I could do was smile pleasantly and continue on to the w.c. where I discovered soon after sitting down, that the light was on a very brief timer and the switch to turn the light back on was out of reach. Knowing what I was in for, maybe that was the reason the men were laughing.

The next day, we set out to explore Amsterdam, a city that brags it has more canals than Venice. It was cold and rainy, but we were enchanted by the narrow cobblestone streets filled with tiny cars, bicycles and motorbikes whizzing around and the old world architecture dating back hundreds of years that wasn't like anything we were familiar with back home.

That evening, we had just finished eating in an Indonesian restaurant when off in the distance, we heard people singing "We Shall Overcome." The lyrics were in Dutch, but the melody of the popular protest song was unmistakable and I wanted to investigate. Following the voices, we came to a large public square filled with young people who looked like college students. Some were singing and carrying placards that we couldn't read. Two boys climbed atop a news kiosk and began fighting. Soon other people, mostly young men, began running every which way and yelling and more fights broke out in the crowd.

What we had thought was a peaceful protest, one we naively hoped might even be against the U.S. involvement in Vietnam, was rapidly becoming violent so we ducked down a narrow side street to escape. A cluster of Dutch policemen with wooden clubs and wicker shields were milling about at the end of the street, looking like they weren't quite sure why they were there. As Bruce and I got closer to them, a crowd of protesters surged down the street so I let go of Bruce's hand and moved off to the side to let them pass. Five policemen descended on me and began beating me around the head and shoulders with their clubs. I screamed, "Stop that! Stop that!" as Bruce rushed to pull me away. Maybe it was my American accent that tipped them off that I wasn't part of the crowd, or maybe they realized five men against one unarmed woman was excessive. At any rate, they stopped beating me and shuffled off without a word of apology.

I wasn't hurt, but I was steaming mad and wanted to register a formal complaint at the American embassy. After I calmed down, I realized the authorities would probably have said it was my own fault for being among the protesters and that would have made me even more angry, so I decided to just consider it part of my sight-seeing experience and laugh it off. In those over-heated days, people our age considered the police to be fascist pigs, anyway.

Soon after we got home, Mark mentioned my experience to one of the reporters at *The News Tribune* where he was working, and to my embarrassment, a story with the lurid title "Bride Beaten in Error" appeared on page 2. Ten years after that, a high school acquaintance said, "Hey, didn't I read you were shot when you were traveling in Europe?"

After Amsterdam, we joined a tour group for a three-day trip down the Rhine, ending in Zurich, Switzerland. From there, we traveled on our own, using our Eurail Passes to get to Bavaria, then traveling through the Austrian Alps to reach Venice, the magical, golden city like no other in the world. We could have been happy staying in Venice for years, but we had only a few days so we rushed around seeing as much as we could in the precious time allotted.

On our second morning in Venice, I bought a copy of the *International Herald Tribune* to get an update on what was happening outside the idyllic world of our honeymoon. Right away I was drawn to an article about a draft board in Ohio that had been bombed by some protesters who were trying to slow down the draft process. The bombing took place in the middle of the night when no one was in the building so there were no casualties, or even minor injuries. However, draft records had been destroyed, possibly saving the lives of countless young men, or at the very least, delaying their induction indefinitely. I was exuberant and rushed to share the good news with Bruce who did not see this act of defiance in the same light as I did. He insisted that taking the law into one's own hands and committing acts of violence is never justified. I protested that no one was hurt, only pieces of paper were destroyed, but still he clung to his belief that people must always follow the law.

Thousands of miles from home, this reckless, unnecessary war had intruded itself into our lives again, or rather, with the foolishness of youth, we had let it intrude itself into our precious time together. Bruce was already classified 1-A and I was sure he would be drafted soon after we returned home. By the spring of 1969, 36,000 American men had already died in Vietnam – 242 in one seven day period in May as documented in *Life Magazine*, and I was very afraid Bruce would be among the dead before the year was over. All I cared about was protecting him and it made me furious that he couldn't accept that sometimes extraordinary steps needed to be taken to save people from the evils of war.

All day, we went back and forth on the subject, when we weren't too angry and sullen to speak at all. That night – a beautiful moonlit night – we had a reservation for a gondola ride on the Grand Canal. With the full moon shimmering on the water and our gondolier singing romantic Italian love songs, we argued the whole time over the relative merits of the selective use of anarchy. At some point that night, we realized we were being silly to fight and wisely decided to avoid the discussion of whether or not anarchy is ever justified for a worthwhile cause. Years later, when people started bombing abortion clinics, Bruce made his point. (In 2009, for our 40th anniversary, we returned to Venice and did it right, and we were even lucky enough to have a full moon.)

Crossing the Atlantic back then took us eight days each way which left us a little more than three weeks to squeeze in as much of Europe as possible so we focused on the highlights – Amsterdam, German cities along the Rhine, Zurich, Munich, Venice, Florence, Rome, the Amalfi Coast, Capri, Naples, Nice and Paris. In every other city, we splurged and got a hotel room with a private bath so we could do our laundry in the sink and hang it over the tub to dry. In Zurich, I was surprised to find the bathroom down the hall was unisex and hot water for the shower was controlled by a coin box. Using an unfamiliar currency, I didn't put enough money in the coin box, causing the water to suddenly shut off mid shampoo. I loved it all.

But, it was over too soon and we had to return home to face Bruce's draft board. Standing on the deck of the Nieuw Amsterdam as the Statue of Liberty came into sight, sadness began to overwhelm me. I wished we could just stay away until the war was over, an impossibility I knew. I also wished I could accept Bruce being drafted with patriotic resignation the way so many other young wives did. But I knew the war was wrong, and it's never right to expect people to passively die for a mistake.

My mother and Bruce's brother Matt met us at the pier. Matt had been monitoring the mail and so far, nothing from the draft board had arrived. At least no one knew we had broken the law and our next hope was that we would continue not hearing anything from the draft board.

However, two weeks later, the notice to report for his physical arrived. Bruce was at work and I was home alone temporarily enjoying my new role as housewife as I prepared my portfolio for a new job search. It was a tense couple of weeks as we tried to prepare ourselves emotionally for what we feared would be inevitable.

Bruce reported to the new federal office building in Newark where military doctors were waiting to examine that day's batch of nervous young men standing in line in their underwear. Bruce had hoped that his chronically low blood pressure might be enough to disqualify him, but anxiety brought his pressure up to a perfect level. Then, the doctor took a look at his feet, which from the standpoint of the infantry, are two of the most important body parts. Bruce was born with hammer toes, a condition that causes the littlest toe on each foot to overlap the one next to it – not a good thing if you might be called upon to march long distances in combat boots. Bruce was sent to another room to be checked out by an orthopedic surgeon – a brilliant saint of a man – who rejected him because a stint in the army with hammer toes might result in a permanent disability and a lifetime military pension. Instead, the doctor gave him a 1Y classification which meant he wouldn't be called up unless the military was desperate.

We celebrated that night with a romantic dinner, a bottle of wine, and the joyous relief that comes when you no longer feel the proverbial angel of death hanging over you. We were free to make our plans for the future, but other young men were forced to continue fighting in Vietnam despite the best efforts of a growing number of anti-war advocates. By 1972, only 30% of Americans still supported the war, but gullible voters believed President Nixon when he declared "peace was at hand" with his "secret plan" to end the war and he was reelected over the peace candidate George McGovern for whom we had worked.

Finally in 1973, President Nixon bowed to public pressure and ended American involvement and started bringing our troops home. For the South Vietnamese, however, the war continued for two more years until their government fell to the communists. By the end of our participation in the war, 58,282 Americans had been killed, 303,644 were wounded and 1,800 were missing in action, never to be seen again.

16

Without the war hanging over us, we could be happy newlyweds. Right away, we took out a mortgage so we could buy out Bruce's brothers' share of the house in Berkeley Heights which was the main part of their parents' estate. This was the house that Bruce had lived in since he was eight-years-old and it was filled with many happy memories. All the trees in the yard, as well as the spring perennials, the flowering shrubs and the rose bushes had been lovingly planted by Bruce's father when he and Jean moved into their first new home back in 1954. There was something very old-fashioned and comforting about our living in the same house where Bruce grew up, surrounded by aunts, uncles and cousins.

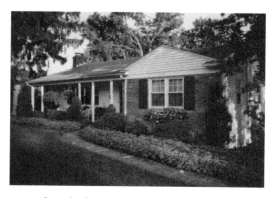

This is the cozy, three-bedroom house in Berkeley Heights where Bruce grew up and where we raised our own children. Matteo Nigro's corn field and a few apple trees had once occupied the space. (Photo by the author)

Bruce's grandfather Matteo Nigro had come to Berkeley Heights from Italy around the turn of the last century and he bought a large house on Springfield Avenue with enough land around it to have a small corn field and a few apple and pear trees, as well as a chicken coop and a barn. He and his wife Giovanna Anastasia were married by proxy while she was still back in their home village of Rionero in Vulture, east of Naples in the Apennine Mountains. I don't know if they had known each other back in Italy or if the marriage was completely arranged by their parents. At any rate, family legend says that he was very disappointed because her nose was so large, but they went on to have six children, plus a few orphaned foster kids that they raised. When each of their children grew up and got married, Matteo gave them a plot of land on which to build their own house. Bruce's father Michael, the first born, was given the plot where Matteo had grown corn, along with one or two apple trees. Bruce's Uncle Ben received the lot next door to Michael's and built a handsome brick house where he and his wife Marge raised their daughters Nancy and Linda. Aunts Tess and Millie and Uncle John were given lots a block away on Lincoln Street where Bruce's cousins John and Saralynne live with their respective families.

This was an entirely new experience for me. I grew up 2,000 miles from my Aunt Mollie and Uncle Harney and his wife Coletta, who I had met only twice in my life. I had cousins on my father's side, but since my mother was estranged from her in-laws, I had never met them and didn't even know their names. Bruce's family welcomed me into their often boisterous, tight-knit clan where everyone talked at once and I had to learn to interrupt, if I was ever going to get a chance to speak. The best part was the food. All the women were great cooks, especially Bruce's mother who I met for the first time when Bruce brought me home to dinner a few months after we met. Bruce's brother's wives were all on diets, but at 110 pounds, I was free to ask for seconds. At this first meeting, his family probably thought I was too quiet to fit into this noisy family, but when I was growing up, my mother was very strict about not interrupting when someone else was speaking. I enjoyed the good Italian food, and as long as my mouth was full, I thought my silence would be acceptable. I just kept eating and before long, his mother was looking in the refrigerator for more food to give me. Good cooks appreciate good eaters so I passed my first test.

Two years after our wedding, Dana Medin was born on June 18, 1971. Because Bruce was one of four boys and his brothers all had boys, we were hoping for a girl and could hardly believe our good fortune in getting a little girl who slept through the night at three weeks old and loved being read to long before she could understand the words. She had big rosy cheeks, brown eyes like Bruce and curly hair. And to make her even more perfect, she started reading before her fourth birthday, which impressed my mother no end. Mom adored her first grandchild and loved buying her clothes and books and taking her to the children's theater productions at the Paper Mill Playhouse.

While I enjoyed being a fulltime mother, I had the nagging feeling that I should be planning for the next stage of my life. Jobs in the field of commercial art were not plentiful and I had long ago accepted that my talent was rather mediocre so I decided, when Dana was three and I was five months pregnant with Jason, that it was

Kbgtkml

time to go back to college. My art school credits were not transferable so I started all over again as a freshman at Rutgers.

By this time, Mark was dating Anne Miller, a woman he was introduced to by their Chinese teacher. Mark had gone back to school to finish his degree at Rutgers and Anne was a senior at St. John's University in New York. After graduation, she had a fellowship to study Chinese at Taiwan University and when she left for her year abroad, Mark was heartbroken. As far as I know, Anne was the first woman Mark had ever loved and he was having a hard time dealing with the separation. He spent hours sitting in his office space down in the basement playing sad love songs on his guitar, driving our mother to distraction. Finally, he couldn't stand being away from her any longer and, with financial help from Mom, he flew to Taiwan to get married in a Chinese ceremony.

By the end of my pregnancy, I could barely squeeze into the student desks at Rutgers. Jason Daniel was born January 17, 1975, right after final exams and two weeks before the start of the spring semester, and he was sleeping through the night at three weeks old. He couldn't have been a more accommodating baby and my mother was delighted to have another grandchild.

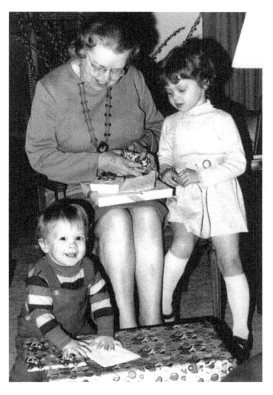

Celebrating Jason's first birthday with Grandma and Dana, (Photo by the author)

Bruce and I loved being parents and we were fortunate not to be burdened with the hardships that my mother and his parents had to endure while they were raising us. It's true that we had to live on a tight budget since I had chosen to be a full-time mother, but we never had to do without anything that was truly important. We had one car and one television, surely enough for one family. Our vacations, when the kids were little, consisted of camping in the Poconos instead of trips to Disney World like most of their friends, or renting a house on Lake Champlain with Mark and Anne for only one week instead of two.

But we still laugh about the time when, over our Pocono camp fire, Bruce accidentally sent his flaming marshmallow flying through the air where it landed on Jay's windbreaker leaving a scorched mess of melting sugar. Or the time when Uncle Mark took them out on Lake Champlain in his inflatable dinghy right before a heavy shroud of fog blew in and then his tiny motor ran out of gas somewhere in the middle of the lake and they had to be towed in. It was scary at the time as I stood on the water's edge waving a high-powered flashlight like a beacon, hoping it would guide them back in, but the incident was good for a nostalgic laugh for all of us many years afterwards. My selective memory has them all wearing life jackets as they set off, but I'm not sure if that's true.

The kids laugh about their early introduction into political activism. When Dana was only three and I was pregnant with Jay, I brought her with me to a supermarket demonstration in support of migrant farm workers. I explained to my innocent little daughter that we were going to picket Pathmark because they were selling nonunion grapes. When we got there, she cheerfully paraded around in front of the store with the other demonstrators, but after about fifteen minutes of this, she grew visibly frustrated and began to yell, "I want some grapes! I want some grapes!" I clapped my hand over her mouth and ushered her away as I realized she thought we were going to *pick* grapes.

Some of Jay's earliest memories involve all of us going to rallies for a nuclear freeze or going door-to-door in support of a freeze referendum on the New Jersey ballot back when President Reagan was recklessly talking about "a limited, winnable nuclear war." By this time, I was the head of the Social Concerns Committee at the Unitarian Church in Summit and our group worked with activists from other local churches to form the Ecumenical Coalition for a Nuclear Freeze. Other childhood memories include demonstrating in front of the Pickatinny Arsenal in north Jersey where nuclear weapons components were made, or going door-to-door canvassing for Walter Mondale and Michael Dukakis when they ran for president. The kids also helped when we sponsored a Vietnamese refugee family at church and when I managed to convince the board to let the Social Concerns Committee join the Interfaith Council for the Homeless.

And the kids still laugh about our dinner time conversations. Remembering my own childhood when my mother, Mark and I read through meals and rarely talked to each other, I wanted my own children to be able to carry on an intelligent conversation on a wide variety of topics. Dana jokes that at any given time, she and Jay were expected to be prepared to discuss nuclear proliferation, Reagan's Star Wars defense system, the death penalty, gun control or the Iran-Contra Affair. Jay added that when other kids were watching sit-coms like "Three's Company," they were watching the MacNeil/Lehrer News Hour on PBS.

I'm so happy that they turned out to be thoughtful, intelligent, well-read adults with empathy for others, a good work ethic and an excellent sense of humor. They appreciate the value of a close-knit family and I am glad we all live close enough that we can get together frequently and even go on vacations together for a week each year.

17

A call before 8:00 a.m. is never a good sign so when the phone rang early on the morning of September 11, 2002, I knew something was wrong. The nurse at Rose Hall said my mother had fallen and was in an ambulance on her way to Overlook Hospital with a suspected broken hip. I finished dressing and rushed over to hospital as they wheeled her into a cubicle in the emergency room where she was quickly evaluated and given a pain killer that added to her mental confusion and only partly masked the pain. As she drifted in and out of consciousness, I waited for the doctors who already had a full schedule of surgeries that morning, placing my mother at the end of the line.

This was the first anniversary of the terrorist attacks on America and ceremonies marking the solemn occasion were being held at Ground Zero in New York, the Pentagon and in a field near Shankesville, Pennsylvania. The mood of the nation was grim as people watched the televised observances of family members reading the names of their loved ones who had died that day. And as fearless and invincible as people tried to appear, the mood was also apprehensive as the nation feared al-Qaeda or some copycat terrorist group would strike again.

By early evening, the surgeon had completed his already scheduled operations and was able to work on my mother's broken hip. He did the best he could on her porous, 92-year-old bones, but a broken hip on a woman her age usually doesn't have a good prognosis. Afterwards, she was moved to a semi-private room where she was hooked up to an IV drip, a catheter, an oxygen tube, a heart monitor, a restraining vest to prevent her from trying to get out of bed, and both arms were tied down to keep her from pulling out the IV. She didn't quite remember where she was or why she was there, but she looked up at me and said, "I'm trying very hard to get used to new things, but I really would prefer going home." If the scene hadn't been so sad, it would have been like one of the ironic *New Yorker* cartoons that my mother had once found so amusing.

I stopped at the hospital each morning on my way to work to see how she was and again on my way home in the evening. In between, I had to hire a "hospital sitter" to stay with her because she probably would have starved to death otherwise. The staff could see that her arms were tied down so she couldn't raise the bed to a sitting position or feed herself, but the food service people would leave her meal tray just out of reach and walk out of the room anyway. And this was a good hospital. I couldn't help wondering what happened to people who didn't have family looking out for them or if they couldn't afford to hire someone to just sit there and tend to their most basic needs.

After a few days, she was moved to a nursing home in Berkeley Heights where she was expected to undergo physical therapy with the stated goal of being able to walk again. But physical therapy was extremely painful and with her severe dementia, she couldn't understand that Medicare would pay for it only if she were making progress.

One evening a priest came by and offered her communion, a ritual she hadn't participated in for at least 65 years, but she opened her mouth to receive the wafer just like the Catholic girl she had once been. Whenever I was there, she wouldn't eat anything but a little ice cream and I worried that her condition would only get worse if she weren't eating a balanced diet. I sought out one of the nurses on duty and told her of my concern. I suppose I shouldn't have been shocked, but it was like a punch in the stomach when the nurse breezed down the hall and, without stopping or tempering her words, tossed over her shoulder, "The body always shuts down near death."

She was three months shy of 93, and we had all watched her slow decline over the past 8 years, and yet hearing that her body was preparing for death stunned me. I moved my mother back to her room at Rose Hall and arranged for Hospice care. They took out her regular bed and brought in a hospital bed and for another two weeks, she slowly got weaker, drifting in and out of sleep.

Then, one Friday afternoon, I got the call at work from the Hospice nurse saying they didn't expect her to last beyond the weekend. I was supposed to work that Saturday, but one of my co-workers quickly agreed to take my place and I prepared to keep a vigil at my mother's bedside.

I had read once that people can hear music even when they are in a coma so I brought my portable CD player and played a variety of her favorite opera arias and show tunes while I passed the time knitting a scarf I had started some time ago and never got around to finishing. The dramatic, tumultuous arias seemed to distress her so I played only the soft, romantic melodies and Celtic folk tunes. When she was awake, she let me moisten her mouth with a wet sponge and she ate some ice cream or pudding from time to time before slipping back into unconsciousness.

Mark, Dana and Jay each came over during the weekend to say goodbye, but she remained unconscious. Bruce spent the day with me on Sunday alternately reading or watching television. By evening, her breathing became more ragged, rousing me from the lethargy I had slipped into. I quickly went to her side and told Bruce to turn off the television. He joined me next to the bed as I stroked her cheek and whispered over and over, "It's OK, you can go now." I don't know why I thought that was the required thing to say, but they were the only words that came to me, and as I stroked her cheek, she quietly breathed her last breath and was gone.

~

When she was in her 80's and still working, she had insisted she didn't want a traditional funeral. She simply wanted to be cremated and the ashes buried next to my father. I managed to get her grudging approval for a small memorial service on the grounds that *we* needed to mark her death in some meaningful way, not just dispose of her body and go on as though nothing had happened.

I delivered the eulogy and Mark, his son Joseph, Dana, Jay, and Bruce all got up to share their memories of her. She had outlived all the ministers who had ever known her and she hadn't attended church in several decades anyway so we didn't bother getting a minister for the service. She would have hated having some clergyman reading notes from an index card and even possibly mispronouncing her name so it was better this way. I was surprised at how many people attended, despite the long drive and torrential rain. The rain was coming down in diagonal sheets making an umbrella almost useless. In fact, when I had woken up the morning of her funeral and saw we weren't just having a shower but a clothes-soaking deluge, I was more than a little dismayed about how this would affect attendance and even the logistics of her internment, but then I remembered New Jersey had been suffering through a bad drought all summer. She would have approved.

Reflections on Visiting My Grandmother
October 2002

Most of all, I remember her books:
Shelves upon dusty shelves of them,
In every room but the bathroom –
Endless escape doors, entranceways
And exits well-worn before I found them.
There were introductions to music and theater,
Records listened to again and again,
Afternoons and evenings under dimmed lights
As the curtain rose upon another realm.
But most of all, she gave me books,
Showed me worlds she loved to visit –
Dorothy in Oz, Anne of Green Gables, The Little Colonel,
Girls who had found adventure and persevered.

In her house, everything was discovery:
The pantry drawers where she stashed
The Thin Mints, the Kraft caramels, the hard candies;
The refrigerator that always held grapes and olives,
Little cans of juice and pints of Haagen-Dazs.
Deviled ham sandwiches served in the dining room

And cheese curls snuck singly from the kitchen.
The displays of objects she culled from catalogs:
Dollhouse furniture, pewter cars, painted plates –
Adult toys to be admired carefully or from afar.
The cable TV box with its rows of buttons
Leading to channels and shows we'd never seen
Before, all marked carefully in her TV Guide.
Her jewelry boxes overflowing with dug-up treasure;
Her puzzles, worked on slowly, over many visits.
The adventure of an attic, ascended to
By narrow stairs, the bare bulb illuminating
Dust motes, we pushed on into dark recesses,
Excavating old toys, old games, lost history.
She saw the potential in Styrofoam
Pieces packed around medical equipment,
Brought them home from the office for us,
For transformation into the space station
Of our imaginings. To house our solar system,
She carved a bright playroom from the dark basement
Out of the trunks and tools, soot and laundry,
The cans and tins of food stacked away – just in case.

Everything in abundance, more than one person
Could need. Security in clutter, in the hoarding
Of things – protection against the days
When there hadn't been enough.
For everything saved, something given –
Piles of school clothes from Morris's,
Where visits lasted hours and all the salespeople
Knew her, and we would run and hide among the racks.
Elaborate Christmas gifts of castles and pirate ships,
Holiday dinners of roast turkey and real gravy,
Formal china and proper manners. Weekend visits
Where we ate sugared cereal, baked cupcakes

And cookies, and let a whole tray run over
Into one giant chocolate chip cookie sheet.

Years later, it was advice – given over and over:
Don't get old. Don't get old. Stressing it,
As if, by saying it often enough, she could
Save us – and maybe she has.
Pay attention, she said. Being old is no fun.
So she got younger – in the process,
Sharing a side we'd never seen before:
The Georgetown Convent student, the Montana child,
A girl who loved teddy bears and picture books.
Looking to please her, we discovered again -
Finding worlds we wouldn't have looked for
Otherwise – new doors to smiles and laughter.
More than anything, I remember her books.

Dana Nigro

~

After suffering the consequences of her father not
having a will and her sisters' profligacy, my mother had
been an astute money manager who managed to squirrel
away a nice sum for Mark and me. I was sad that she
hadn't enjoyed herself more while she was young enough
to travel. Her last trip had been the one she and I took
driving around the southwest for three weeks just before
Bruce and I got married. She did like going to the theater
so the two of us saw some operas in New York and had
season tickets to McCarter Theater in Princeton and to
the Paper Mill Playhouse where I had worked for ten
years as the publicist. But her friends had all died off

or moved away and she was not good at making new friends so when we were not together, I'm afraid she was very lonely.

There must have been many things she regretted not doing when she was younger: she didn't go to college and she hadn't traveled to the far-away places she had read about, but if there were other regrets, she never really talked about them. I wish I had asked her what she would have majored in if she had been able to go to college. Her interests were so eclectic, judging by the wide range of subjects in her enormous collection of books, that I can't even venture a guess. But circumstances had forced her always to take the practical route so she probably would have said it was pointless to speculate on "might have beens" and just take pride in what she had accomplished despite the obstacles.

The only hint she gave that she might have done some things differently was when she cautioned that I should never spend the principle, only the interest, but then added that I should not forgo the opportunity of doing something if it is really *very* important to me or I might regret it for the rest of my life. With those words in mind, I used part of my inheritance to fulfill my lifelong dream of having my very own boat.

When I was fifteen, I used to ask my mother to drive me to Raritan Bay so I could look at the boats at the yacht club. With the certainty that only teenagers can have, I planned to have a schooner when I grew up and I was going to sail it all over the world. She would indulge me by driving all the way to Perth Amboy and waiting patiently while I admired all the beautiful sail boats moored at the mouth of the Raritan River. I fantasized about which one I would buy when I became a rich artist and she listened without once saying, "Don't be ridiculous! Do you realize how much a boat like that would cost and you'd need a whole crew to operate it. You'll never be able to afford a row boat, let alone a sail boat like one of those!"

At the time, I was too young and naïve even to realize she was probably exercising amazing restraint in not pouring cold water all over my dream. After all, her own life had been a succession of deflated dreams, but she let me continue believing that in my own future everything was possible. When the time finally came, I bought a more manageable 25 foot cabin cruiser, not a schooner after all, and I named it *The Eileen O'Meara*.

Mark, on the other hand, was intensely practical and used part of his inheritance to buy a ten-year-old car that was only a modest improvement over the one he had been driving. Sometime over the years, he had turned into an ascetic who believed strongly in repairing and reusing everything rather than succumbing to the urge to buy new. I tried arguing that if everyone lived by that philosophy, the world economy would fall apart, but he didn't agree. He had inherited our father's self-reliant ability to build or repair just about anything he needed and if he couldn't, then he just did without. More and more, he seemed to be defiantly doing without. He also hadn't been to the dentist or eye doctor in more than a decade.

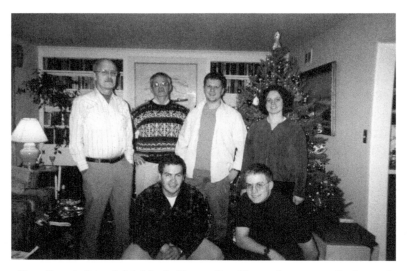

Standing, left to right: Mark, Bruce, Jay, Dana; front row: Carlos and Joseph. (Photo by the author)

Originally, Mom's plan was for Mark to inherit her house in Metuchen, but by this time, he didn't really have the energy to take good care of his own house in North Bergen which was close to his job at *The Record* so he agreed that it was too impractical for him to own two houses. He and Anne were separated but living just a few blocks apart so that Joseph could be close to both his parents.

I was running errands one day when my cell phone rang. I pulled off the highway to take the call from Mark who wanted to tell me about Joseph's upcoming theatrical production at the magnet high school where he was a senior. Mark adored his son and was understandably proud of all his achievements. I told him that we would be there to hear Joseph sing and then Mark added what must have been his real reason for calling, "I have stage four lung cancer."

He probably was afraid I would scream, "We told you so! We've all been begging you to stop smoking for years! You know bad lungs run in the family." But I certainly would never have been cruel enough to say what he clearly already knew.

Over the next several months, Anne, Joseph and I formed a team: Joseph checked on his father every day and brought over food; Anne took care of the insurance paperwork and I took Mark to his weekly chemotherapy appointments at Hackensack University Medical Center. My empathetic boss at the Community FoodBank let me take off every Wednesday afternoon to help Mark. First, we went to his favorite diner for lunch and then drove across town to the hospital. While he was hooked up to the IV, he calmly did *The New York Times* crossword puzzle and then we drove over to Anne's house, overlooking the Hudson River, where the three of us had dinner and Mark filled her and Joseph in on the latest prognosis. As we sat around the dining room table sharing a meal, flashes of Mark's old sense of humor would come through, despite the ordeal he was enduring, and I loved these rare and very fleeting moments of being a cohesive family again.

One time, he was talking about feeding the mice that had set up a nest in his house. I exclaimed, "You feed the mice, too? How did we end up this way?" And we both laughed with more than a little touch of melancholy. Our mother loved pets, but she was a ruthless killer of bugs and anything deemed to be vermin. If a fly or bee was beating itself against the window, trying desperately to get outside where it knew it belonged, Mom would spray it with Raid until the poor thing was just a puddle of foam and then she'd beat it with the fly swatter for another minute or so, just to make sure. At a very young age, I began to side with the bugs and begged her to let me take care of getting them out of the house. Then, I'd put a glass over the helpless thing, slide an envelope underneath and usher the bug outside. Mom thought I was being ridiculous, but she didn't interfere.

His cancer was inoperable, but the various drugs could keep him alive for an undetermined amount of time. I didn't like Mark's doctor. He had a stony coldness about him and I urged Mark to at least seek a second opinion, but he was resigned to his prognosis and accepted it without complaint. I wanted him to fight harder, but he must have realized he had been seriously ill for a long time because he had had a persistent cough and was always tired. And yet he didn't have a regular doctor and was still smoking his favorite cigars. It infuriated me that every Wednesday, before going to the hospital for his chemotherapy, he'd slowly walk around the corner to the neighborhood bodega to buy The New York Times, for the crossword puzzle, and several packs of cigars.

"Why are you still smoking?" I hissed with barely suppressed rage.

"If I stop smoking, will I live?" he asked.

I had to admit that he might not live longer, but if he stopped irritating his lungs further, making it more difficult to breathe, at least the quality of his remaining time would be better. For years, Anne had begged him to stop smoking because she didn't want him to die young like our father did. Mark just felt she was nagging him and tuned it out, which was one of the factors leading to the dissolution of their marriage. She must have felt, as I did, that Mark's addiction made him choose tobacco over the people who loved him, something we both could not understand.

Mark realized his goal of living long enough to see Joseph graduate from high school in June of 2005, but by then he was deathly pale and walked like an old man. That August, the heat was unbearable and Mark didn't have air conditioning in his house. Then, suddenly, Peter Jennings, a TV journalist who Mark respected, died of lung cancer and Mark's condition rapidly deteriorated.

Bruce and I brought him to live with us because he was too weak to live alone any longer. A week later, after being up all night thinking, he told me he had decided to discontinue the chemotherapy. I had to respect the decision that only he could make, and yet it was hard watching him give up. To make him more comfortable, we rented a hospital bed, brought in Hospice and hired a live-in home health aide to look after him while I was at work. Joseph came over frequently to visit, and when Mark was feeling strong enough, the two of them would sit out on the front porch to talk. Mark was anxious to share as many anecdotes from his life as he could recollect and Joseph diligently took notes.

When he couldn't sleep, it comforted him to sit on the porch, in the dark, listening to the repetitive din of the crickets and watching for nocturnal animals. One night, a small herd of deer wandered through the yard, paused to look at him sitting so still, and then continued on their way. During the day, a chipmunk ran right over his foot on its way to gather up the bird seed and peanuts I had thrown out that morning, and every afternoon, a hummingbird came to feed from the impatiens hanging nearby. These simple pleasures delighted him and made me happy that we had insisted on his coming to stay with us.

One evening, Mark asked me if I'd like to sit on the porch with him and talk, but he was smoking yet another cigar and I stubbornly declined. Now I sadly regret being so judgmental about his smoking and missing my last chance to ask him what else he could remember about our parents or stories he had heard about our other ancestors.

By mid-September, he was too weak to get out of bed, and most telling of all, he no longer craved tobacco. The Hospice nurse gave him oral syringes of morphine that he could squirt into his mouth whenever the pain or anxiety became too much to bear. He didn't have much of an appetite for balanced meals, but we were encouraged one evening when the phone rang as Bruce, the aide, and I were eating dinner in the kitchen. It was Mark calling on his cell phone wanting to know if we had any cherry vanilla ice cream. "Coming right up," I said, as Bruce put down his fork and rushed to the store to stock up on Mark's favorite flavors of ice cream.

We were hoping he would rally and live for a few more months because Jay and Deané were getting married on October 23rd, but it wasn't to be. As he got weaker, Mark told me that he didn't want us sitting around him keeping a deathbed vigil. He had always been a very private person and he wanted to be allowed to die alone, with dignity. During the night, I checked on him periodically, and then left the room. Very early in the morning of October 7th, I went in his room to see how he was doing and heard the unmistakable gurgling sound in his throat. I went back to bed and lay there waiting. Around 5:00 a.m., I returned to his room and found that he had stopped breathing. Then, I gently closed his eyes, just as I had done for our mother exactly three years and one day earlier.

Also like our mother, he was adamant about not wanting a traditional funeral. He had asked to be cremated and wanted me to scatter his ashes in the Shark River where he used to go fishing many years ago. I suggested Lake Champlain, instead, because we had all shared happy times there when the kids were young and he and Anne and Joseph were still together. Mark liked that idea so the following June, we rented a lakeside house big enough for all eight of us, as well as Jay and Deané's dog Arnie, and spent a week simply being a family that enjoyed each other's company. I had brought my mother's ashes, too, - - the ones I had originally intended to scatter from a mountain overlooking Butte, but I liked our new plan better.

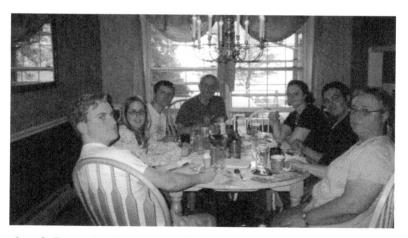

Joseph, Deane, Jay, Bruce, Dana, Carlos and Anne sharing a meal together after scattering Mark's and Mom's ashes. (Photo by the author)

One afternoon, we rented a boat and sailed out to the middle of the lake, and as we each shared a special memory of Mark, Joseph scattered his father's ashes while I sprinkled my mother's on top, mingling their shared

DNA in a milky cloud that floated off and gradually sank to the bottom of the lake. My mother wasn't a sentimental woman, but I think even she would have found a certain poetic beauty in being there with her son.

18

Jay and Deané's wedding on October 23, 2005 was a beautiful and very happy occasion. True, it was only 16 days after Mark's death, but his suffering was over and he had made it clear that he didn't want his passing to cast a pall over their nuptials. I think in the old days, the wedding would have been canceled and the family would have been in mourning for a year, but fortunately we live in a time that honors the dead while respecting that life must be allowed to go on for those left behind.

The ceremony was outside in the garden of the English Manor, and despite a chill in the autumn air, the sun was shining brightly and the mood was joyous. The next day, they left for Italy and Dubrovnik, two places that figure prominently in our family's history.

Jay and Deané had met at least 8 years before while they were both at Rutgers, but didn't start dating until a few years after graduation when they reconnected at a Halloween party. By this time, Jay was working in financial services and Deané was an attorney at a Newark law firm, a job she hated because the long hours didn't allow for much of a life outside of work. With her background as a civil engineer in addition to law, she was able to find a new job tailor-made for her at an international engineering company that sends her all over the world as a project manager with strong negotiating skills. Jay is a vice president at Morgan Stanley in New

York's financial district and does something involved with preventing obscenely wealthy people from engaging in insider trading. She earns more than he does which Jay finds very liberating, a sure sign that he is a confident man well-adapted for the new age of strong, professional women.

They bought a three-bedroom house in Verona with a nice backyard for their two rescued dogs. Their black lab Arnie needed a playmate so they adopted a white boxer they named Nori, after the Antinori Winery in Tuscany where Dana had arranged for them to have lunch and a private tour on their honeymoon.

Nine years later, the whole family was filled with joy when, through the miracle of in vitro fertilization, the twins Matteo and Lara were born, adding one more generation to our combined family lineage.

Dana is a senior editor at *Wine Spectator Magazine* and managing editor of *Wine Spectator Online*. In early 2001, one of her co-workers introduced her to his best friend Carlos Colomer who had just moved to New York from New Orleans to start a job at *The New York Times* as a copy editor with their online edition. His friend had good instincts as a matchmaker because they fell in love and a few months later, Carlos moved into Dana's Weehawkin apartment.

Carlos is an avid reader and loves talking politics so he fit right in with our family. He even took up scuba diving because Dana loved the sport which she had taken up after suffering too many injuries horseback riding.

Ad revenues were down at *The New York Times*, resulting in Carlos being laid off. Eventually, he landed a job as a copy editor on the sports desk at *The Record*, the paper where Mark worked, and when Mark became too ill to continue working, Carlos moved to the news desk. As of this writing, Carlos found his dream job as a copy editor for *The New Yorker* online and is one of the few people who truly loves going to work.

Finally, the day that Bruce and I, as well as Carlos' parents, had been praying for arrived – Dana and Carlos were married. We had a lovely ceremony and reception at Bretton Woods in Morris Plains, with one of my advocacy colleagues officiating. Carlos' three-year-old niece was a delightful flower girl who really warmed to her role once she got over her initial wariness. The next day, the newlyweds left for a honeymoon in Italy and Dubrovnik where they visited the nearby island of Korcula, site of a tiny church with the Medin coat of arms on the wall.

The following year, Joseph graduated from Montclair State University where he had majored in theater arts. While there, he met and fell in love with Caitlin Orvetz, one of his classmates, and a few months after graduation they were married.

Dana and Carlos bought a house just a mile from the family home where she grew up, adopted one of my foster cats that they named Mignon, and planned to start a family of their own.

After one miscarriage and several years of disappointment, Dana and Carlos were blessed with another IVF miracle when Gabriel was born. Gabriel and the twins are only two-and-a-half years apart, and it is my hope that they will grow up to be close friends who cherish the bonds of family and lots of shared memories of good times together.

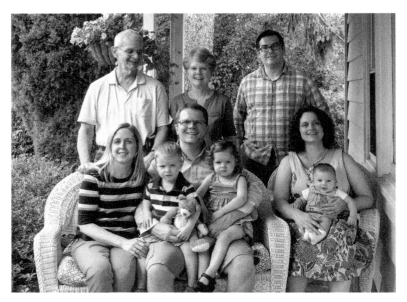

Top, left to right: Bruce & Meara Nigro, Carlos Colomer; seated: Deané, Matteo, Jay & Lara Nigro, Dana & Gabriel Colomer. (Photo by Deané Nigro)

~

In 2010, Bruce and I retired. His parents had died young and never had the opportunity to travel or pursue activities other than working. My mother feared having nothing to do all day and being isolated at home so she kept on working until she was 84 and then was too old and frail to travel on her own. She hadn't cultivated any interests beyond working and reading, and then, sadly, her vision and increasing dementia made it difficult to do either.

By the time Bruce retired, he had worked his way up from case worker to Director of the Essex County Division of Welfare, one of the largest welfare departments in the country, and was highly respected for how well he ran an agency of 800 people with an annual budget of over $70 million. Even advocacy groups representing low-income people in the state respected him because they knew he cared about the clients and put their needs first. He also served for several years as president of the New Jersey Welfare Directors Association and under his leadership, relations between the county government agencies and the advocacy community became more of a partnership with shared goals rather than an adversarial relationship.

After being a stay-at-home mom for 12 years while the kids were young and I was working on my bachelor's degree at Rutgers, I was hired by the Paper Mill Playhouse as a publicist. It wasn't a great-paying job, but what it lacked in financial reward, it made up for in pure enjoyment. Many years earlier, my mother had taken me to shows at the Paper Mill and I had grown up on the musicals and old-fashioned operettas that the Playhouse was known for. I loved the excitement of performance days and getting to know the actors when I took them out to lunch or dinner with feature writers from the newspapers. Theater staff used to joke that by the time these performers were at the Paper Mill, they were either on their way up in their careers or on their way down, but they were all professional Equity actors and most of them were friendly, very talented and fun to be with.

I think of this as the glamorous faze of my life when I attended opening night parties, black tie galas at the Hilton and took actors to elegant 4-star restaurants in New York. For my birthdays and Christmas, Mom enjoyed taking me shopping at Morris Stores in Metuchen to outfit me with dresses and accessories appropriate for the new role I was playing.

Many of the actors and most of the artistic staff at the theater were gay, a part of society I had never been around before except briefly at art school, and I loved getting to know them as friends. Growing up as a shy little girl in predominately white, heterosexual Metuchen, I had been exposed to a very limited world. This was a new experience and I loved it.

But after almost ten years, it suddenly came to an end when the theater was near bankruptcy because the artistic director habitually ran over budget and fund raising was down because of competition from the New Jersey Performing Arts Center which was about to open in Newark. Several people on the staff were tossed overboard, and I was looking for a new job.

By fortuitous coincidence, the Community Foodbank of New Jersey, the state's largest charity providing donated food to over 1,000 programs serving the poor, was looking for a director of communications and advocacy. While the Paper Mill Playhouse job was fun, it didn't really satisfy that part of me that wanted to be doing something socially relevant.

When I was hired, my co-workers told me to stock up on long underwear and warm socks, and a pair of knee-high rubber boots was a definite necessity for the days when it rained. The Foodbank's 280,000 square foot warehouse, a former Kraft manufacturing plant, was located in an artificial bowl created in the 1950's when tons of earth were dug out and hauled over to Newark to expand the airport. The warehouse was at the end of Evans Terminal, a street so ugly it looked like a movie set for a film about the seedy underworld. Whenever it rained hard, water poured down the street and from the cliff behind the warehouse creating a moat around the building. We had to park our cars up the street and wade carefully through the filthy water, but when it was over our knees, they ferried us in by truck. I was enchanted by it all.

I especially liked the people I worked with, all of whom were there because they wanted to help people who were so poor they couldn't meet their most basic need for food. The organization was committed to giving jobs to former offenders and addicts in recovery, many of the people who were most apt to be at soup kitchens or emergency pantries. More than half of my colleagues were felons or former drug addicts and I loved talking politics with them and helping them register to vote once they had completed their parole.

My favorite part of my job was advocacy. I relished the challenge of meeting with members of Congress or their aides and trying to persuade them that federal nutrition programs, as well as other key parts of the social safety net, were essential for the well-being of a significant segment of our population.

When Jon Corzine, former CEO of Goldman Sachs, was elected to the U.S. Senate, he brought his teenage son to the FoodBank for a day of volunteering. Usually, when politicians showed up to volunteer, it was strictly a photo op and after the media left, the politicians were out the door. But Senator Corzine specifically requested that the media not be notified. He just wanted to spend the day working on a project with his son without making a big fuss about it, so he donned a hairnet and spent several anonymous hours repackaging noodles. Back in Washington a few months later, he met with our little group of anti-hunger advocates for almost an hour to talk about legislation, something senators rarely ever do.

A few years later, when he was New Jersey's governor, he created a $6 million line item in the budget for the State Food Purchase Program to help food banks buy the nutritious foods that are rarely donated.

One day, famous rock legend Bruce Springsteen called my boss Kathleen and said he'd like to see the facility. He was a longtime financial supporter of the FoodBank since its beginning in a former meat packing plant in Newark, but he had never been to the new, much larger warehouse in Hillside. Usually big rock stars travel with an entourage, but Bruce drove up by himself in an old pickup truck, dressed in jeans, a faded jacket and a Dolphins baseball cap. We had a large group of teenage volunteers that day, but no one recognized him out of context walking around the warehouse. On stage, he's a flamboyant performer, but in person, he seems almost shy. Kathleen and I took him around the warehouse to meet the staff and everyone wanted their picture taken with him. He graciously posed with everyone while I snapped away, and I regret to this day that I didn't ask someone to take my picture with him. He stayed and ate lunch with students in our food service training program, most of whom were welfare-to-work moms or men recently out of jail or drug treatment.

After a meeting of anti-poverty advocates I spoke at in Trenton was written up in most of the state's newspapers, an article about the challenges activists face appeared in *The Asbury Park Press,* Bruce Springsteen's home town paper. He wrote a letter to the editor in which he criticized Governor Christie's push to lower taxes for the wealthy while simultaneously cutting state spending on programs to help the poor. He praised the work being done by the anti-poverty community and mentioned me by name, along with several of my colleagues.

A major part of my job description included publicizing the Foodbank's programs to help low-income families. We had recently opened two Kids Cafés in Hudson County where the child poverty rate was over 25%. These cafés provide free dinners to poor kids in already existing after-school programs and every effort is made to provide nutritious foods that are familiar to children of different ethnic backgrounds.

A reporter from *The Jersey Journal* interviewed me about the program and I was quoted in the article describing a typical menu for the predominantly Hispanic population at that Kids Café. A few days later, Rush Limbaugh, the right-wing TV and radio provocateur ridiculed me and the whole concept of the Kids Café program. He scoffed at the idea that there were any hungry children in New Jersey, despite the Census statistics and likened the ethnic menus that I had described to preposterous things like toad livers and fried newt tongues. I was furious, and utterly amazed, that anyone would be cruel enough to disparage a program that helps poor, defenseless children. I can understand that some people feel entitled to criticize low-income adults for whatever shortcomings they think are responsible for their condition. But little children? The more I thought about it, the more angry I became until my blood pressure was the highest it's ever been. I only know that because I had an appointment that afternoon to get a tetanus booster, and the nurse took my blood pressure. She was a little surprised that it was 145 over 90 when it's normally about 120 over 70. So I recounted the whole Rush Limbaugh story just before the doctor came in, and when he checked my blood pressure again a few minutes later, it had risen a few notches to 148 over 90.

Rush Limbaugh gets paid millions to cater to a particular segment in this country. Republican politicians bow down before him because a critical remark from him can ruin their careers. At times, his comments have been so offensive that hundreds of companies have felt compelled to stop advertising on his show and yet, he is sometimes considered the de facto head of the Republican Party.

In 2014, Bruce and I each went to our fiftieth high school reunions. My reunion committee asked everyone to sum up what we had been doing for the past fifty years in 100 words or less, which is no small feat. It was then I realized that two of the things I am most proud of in my professional life were being personally ridiculed by Rush Limbaugh for promoting programs that help poor children and praised by Bruce Springsteen, a rock icon with compassion, who has helped raise more than $6.5 million for over 500 anti-poverty organizations in the United States.

~

Bruce and I are determined to enjoy our later years so with his pension and my 401K, along with our investments that we were able to make by living within our means all these years, and with the money my mother left me, we are able to travel, and pursue a wide variety of interests. Bruce has been studying Italian for several years, and while his accent is terrible, his vocabulary is excellent and he has managed to make himself understood during our trips to Italy to visit the little villages where his ancestors were born.

I take painting classes at the Summit Art Center, as well as free classes through Union County College. I've always loved animals so I volunteer with a cat rescue group. Bruce and I used to foster homeless cats to socialize them in preparation for adoption, but we ended up keeping so many of them that we had to stop at seven.

As part of my continuing search for connection to family, we visited Denmark and Norway where my father's family originated. Bruce and I didn't know what towns they came from or if there are any relatives still living in either country. It was more of an emotional journey just to absorb a feeling of where my ancestors had once lived. That was enough and I was satisfied.

EPILOGUE

I wonder if my mother ever thought about all the amazing changes that she lived to see. Probably her generation witnessed more life-changing technological innovations in a relatively short period of time than any other before or after. When she was born in 1910, her parents still rode around in a horse-drawn carriage replaced soon afterwards by one of the very early automobiles that required a hand crank to get the motor running. Her father even broke his arm trying to get his first car started and cautioned the children not to tell their mother, as if she wouldn't have noticed.

As a child in Butte, her family had a telephone in their home as well as a phonograph, but both were still considered luxuries by most Americans. It was the rapid growth of new methods of electronic communication, as well as the spread of indoor plumbing to the middle class, both of which required enormous quantities of copper, that brought her father John O'Meara to Butte in the first place. Without the need for men to mine the precious ore, perhaps he would have stayed back in Bunmahon and become a farmer, changing the course of our family history completely. Had gold and silver not been discovered out west, perhaps Marco Medin would have remained back in Dalmatia continuing the family's fruit export business among the markets of Europe. If the British had not oppressed their Irish subjects, perhaps the

Thorntons would have stayed in Ballinrobe and Sarah would never have ended up in Virginia City, Nevada, where she met Marco. It's fascinating to think of all the "what ifs" – all the historical twists of fate that ultimately led the creation of each of us.

My mother lived to see the evolution of telephones from the first wire-dependent, operator-assisted versions to the rise of wireless cell phones, and the old crank-up record player with the bell-shaped amplifier from her childhood grew up to be a stereo sound system combined with an AM/FM radio. Mom bought her first black & white television in 1956 which she replaced with a color console by 1970. With the advent of cable TV, she had more channels than she knew what to do with and had to bookmark her *TV Guide* so she could keep track of all the options. By the time she had a VCR and a DVD player, her eye sight was failing, and all the tiny black buttons on the black boxes began to intimidate her. Mark's offer to have two-year-old Joseph show her how to operate her latest gadgets did not relieve her exasperation.

In the world of medicine, she was born at a time when infants, including two of her brothers, died from diphtheria and other childhood ailments that were largely eradicated by the time Mark and I were born. Fifty million people world-wide had died from the flu pandemic that ravaged her family in 1918, but advances in diagnosis and treatment since then mean that pandemics can be brought under control before they have a chance to spread all over the world. Medical research into the human genome and the development of new diagnostic tools added dramatically to the life spans of average people. And, most meaningful to our family, new knowledge and techniques in the field of fertility treatments brought us our three precious miracles: Matteo, Lara and Gabriel.

Much as I would like to, I can't avoid mentioning the technological changes to warfare that occurred in my mother's lifetime. When she was a child, war was still a horrific event, but for the most part, fighting was conducted on a battlefield and weapons were still confined to bullets and bombs, except for the despicable use of mustard gas and other chemical poisons that were occasionally used by combatants despite international laws prohibiting them. The invention of nuclear weapons during World War II, however, changed the political dynamics between nations forever.

In 1925, when she traveled from Butte, Montana to boarding school in Washington, D.C., it took three days to travel by train. By the time my father was dying in 1947, she flew to Montana in an airplane with propellers and by 1968 when Aunt Mollie died, she flew back to Butte in a jet.

The first movies she saw as a child were jerky, silent black &white films and before long, she was enjoying musical extravaganzas in full Technicolor on a giant screen. Movie theaters were also a refuge from the oppressive heat and humidity people had to endure before air conditioning became commonplace. The Carrier Engineering Corporation invented the first cooling systems in 1915 and by 1925, movie theaters were installing the systems all over the country. When Mark and I were children in the 1950's, Mom would sometimes take us to escape the heat at a Forum Theater double feature, and then we'd have dinner at the equally-frigid Duchess Diner. It didn't matter that some of the movies weren't really appropriate for young children. A few blissful hours in a climate-controlled environment were all that mattered. Eventually, Mom had a few window air conditioners installed, but she didn't like the noise and rarely turned them on.

Full-service supermarkets were just coming into their own in the 1950's. Before the new A&P in Metuchen was built, I can still remember accompanying my mother into the old one with sawdust on the creaky wooden floor, a large pickle barrel by the old cash register, and housewives had to ask the store clerk for the items they wanted to purchase because everything was out of reach behind the counter. We had an electric refrigerator, but for as long as I can remember, she still referred to it as "the ice box" from her childhood days when the ice man would deliver a huge block of ice to keep the food from spoiling.

She didn't hesitate a minute to embrace whatever time-saving gadgets came along to make housework easier from dishwashers to clothes dryers, power mowers to snow blowers.

She loved her electric, self-correcting typewriter at work which was so much easier to use than her old finger-pounding manual Underwood, but she hated computers and was sure they were only a passing fad. Because of this, she missed out on the awe-inspiring wonders of the internet that I think she would have appreciated if she had only given it a chance.

But what I remember most about my mother's adjustment to a rapidly changing world was her total fascination with space travel. On July 20, 1969, Neil Armstrong and Buzz Aldrin were the first American astronauts to land on the moon, and because much of the voyage would be televised, my mother and Mark came over to our house to see it on our color TV. The world watched in awe for hours as the astronauts, thousands of miles away, talked with Mission Control in Houston in preparation for the much-anticipated moon walk. Finally, around 2 a.m. eastern time, Neil Armstrong climbed down from the space capsule, stepped onto the lunar surface to begin his famous walk and said, "That's one small step for a man, one giant leap for mankind."

Bruce, Mark and I were struggling to stay awake to appreciate this historic moment while my mother was wired with unwavering attention. She was sitting on the edge of her chair, leaning forward with laser focus so as not to miss any of the slightly hazy lunar images on the TV screen. She knew this was momentous and she wasn't taking even one minute of it for granted.